"A lovely spiritual guide to help you live a more radiant life, inside and out."

Sophie Uliano, *New York Times* best-selling author of *Gorgeously Green*

"I love nothing more than to make women feel powerful, great about themselves and their body. *The Radiant Woman's Handbook* by Joanna Runciman, is yet another inspiring book that can help to move women forward into their goodness and greatness! In my opinion now is the time for the culture of women to step up, step in, and find their radiance."

Debbie Rosas, Co-creator and founder of the Nia Technique®

"In *The Radiant Woman's Handbook,* Joanna provides a very personal and pragmatic approach to a healthier and happier lifestyle."

Bruce Lourie, co-author of *Slow Death by Rubber Duck*

"*The Radiant Woman's Handbook* should really be every woman's new best friend! This warm, wise and inspired blueprint to a genuinely healthy and happy life will leave you glowing, naturally, from the inside out."

Adria Vasil, author of *EcoHolic* and *EcoHolic Body*

"Sensible advice written in a readily accessible manner."

Bruce Blumberg, PhD., Professor Depts. of Developmental and Cell Biology and Pharmaceutical Sciences, University of California

"Joanna's holistic approach to living a radiant life is inspiring. Her book provides easy to implement strategies to improve all aspects of your life, to eliminate toxics (whether emotional or physical), and to be simply more joyfully radiant."

Jennifer Taggart, TheSmartMama.com

Y0-BFE-911

"In *The Radiant Woman's Handbook* Joanna provides practical words of wisdom with a depth of knowledge and science to back it up. The wisdom of a grandmother's words, a scientist's scrutiny for proof and a coach's (or counsellor's) encouragement for self discovery wrapped into a beautifully written book.

Thank you for encouraging women everywhere to leap into their radiance and to continue leaping forward on that journey. The book is an enjoyable and insightful read that led me to reflect personally on my own journey to radiance."

Dr. Shannon Patterson, owner of The Adjusting Room

The Radiant Woman's Handbook

Sensible, positive solutions
for reducing toxins and loving your body

. . .

Joanna Runciman

. . .

With all best
wishes
Joanna

ACTUAL ORGANICS PRESS

The Radiant Woman's Handbook:
Sensible, Positive Solutions for Reducing Toxins and Loving Your Body
First Edition Trade Book, 2013
Copyright © 2013 by Joanna Runciman

Library and Archives Canada Cataloguing in Publication

Runciman, Joanna, author
    The radiant woman's handbook : sensible, positive solutions for reducing toxins
    and loving your body / by Joanna Runciman.

Includes bibliographical references and index.
ISBN 978-0-9919495-0-2 (pbk.)
1. Women--Health and hygiene. 2. Beauty, Personal. 3. Women--
Nutrition. 4. Organic living. I. Title.

RA778.R86 2013   613.04244   C2013-904734-4

Scripture quotations, unless otherwise indicated, are from **THE MESSAGE**, copyright © by Eugene H. Peterson 1993, 1994, 1995, 1996, 2000, 2001, 2002 and used by permission of NavPress Publishing Group.

To order more copies of *The Radiant Woman's Handbook* please contact: www.actualorganics.com.

Editor: Arlyn Lawrence, Gig Harbor, WA
Book Design: Brianna Showalter, Ruston, WA
Cartoons: Sarah Leigh, Vancouver, Canada. Photography: SusanCarmody.com
Proof Reading: David Darling, Vancouver, Canada.
Printed in the U.S.A.

Disclaimer: The information contained in this book is intended as a general guide only and does not relate to any particular individual or circumstance. It is not intended to constitute medical or other advice. Neither the author nor the publishers can be held responsible for claims arising from the inappropriate use of any remedy or exercise regime. Neither the author nor the publisher make any claim in relation to the suitability or efficacy of any information in this book for any particular individual or circumstance. Do not attempt self-diagnosis or self-treatment for any conditions before consulting a medical professional or qualified practitioner. Do not begin any exercise programme or undertake any self-treatment whilst taking other prescribed drugs, receiving therapy or suffering from any injury or illness without first seeking professional guidance. Always seek specialist and specific medical or other advice before making changes to your diet or lifestyle. Publisher and author expressly disclaim any liability to the reader of the book.

Table of Contents

· Foreword ·

There can never be too many guides helping us navigate the world of synthetic chemicals, harmful food pesticides and toxic cosmetics. Complex and unapproachable technical studies abound, dozens of detox fads are advertised, yet only a smattering of books are available that offer genuine guidance to concerned consumers. In *The Radiant Woman's Handbook*, Joanna provides a very personal and pragmatic approach to a healthier and happier lifestyle.

As with many people I have come across, through my research and international speaking engagements, Joanna's story begins with overcoming her personal struggles and her encounters with ineffective treatments with synthetic chemicals.

Joanna recognizes that beauty is far more than skin deep and provides thoughtful insights into appreciating what we have around us. Life is more than an accumulation of material wealth. There is a spiritual element to our lives that Joanna embraces fully and correctly credits with our general state of well-being.

Yet she does not ignore the fact that there is an important element of beauty in our skin and to this end devotes much of her book to healthy, organic lifestyle choices that offer simple and sensible alternatives to the otherwise toxic personal care products we are being sold.

And finally, Joanna's story is one of hope, happiness and helpfulness. These are all things that we are very much in need of these days.

Bruce Lourie, best-selling co-author *Slow Death by Rubber Duck*
Toronto
May 2013

· Introduction ·

If asked, most women will come up with something they would like to change about their bodies. They would like to: "Look younger", "lose ten pounds", "have longer hair", "have nicer feet", or "have whiter teeth". Yet the reality is that if those things were actually changed, that feeling of "something missing" would likely remain.

So, what are women really searching for? I believe it is radiance. This book can help you find radiance—and it certainly is not in a $150 pot of face cream, regardless of the elaborate claims on the attractive packaging. I wrote this book to show you how to care for yourself with a different approach than you'll find in most self-help beauty guides on the market today. I hope this book helps you love your body—to think about it not in the sense of what's wrong that you want to improve but rather what is wonderful that you want to nurture and protect.

I want to give you sensible suggestions that fit into your busy life. You may find life gets less hectic when you adopt some of them. You will master methods for living a more radiant and less toxic life.

Over the past twelve years I have made significant changes in my life that led me to where I am today, sharing with you what I have learnt during my honours degree, chef's training, Nia belts, life coaching course, and research. My varied reading and education has allowed me to make connections that lead to a natural approach to be radiant.

I want to show you how to navigate the vast array of information on health and wellness, beauty and skin care aimed at women today. Is it just me that feels it is relentless? Learning how to live near it without being consumed by it is a first step to radiant living. This book will start you on that path.

I live in British Columbia with my husband and dog. I feel fortunate to have an impact on women's lives through writing my blog and articles for a local newspaper as well as giving presentations in Canada and in my home country, England. I share recipes and simple ways to reduce the amount of synthetic chemicals you meet in skin care and the environment with an aim to looking and feeling radiant.

This book addresses the many popular questions I am often asked: "What skin care is good?", "How can I look after my skin as I grow older?", "What do you eat to keep well?", "How do you make time for yourself?" It might surprise you, as I am not advocating kale smoothies and rigorous exercise regimes. I like kale but I also like balance. I propose we start to be kind to ourselves—the eating well comes out of love and a desire to care for our bodies.

I wish to encourage women to live to their full potential, radiantly and joyfully. Having read the book you will have the tools you need to regain your inner glow and enjoy being the woman you are. We are all different in very beautiful ways and this book celebrates that.

By reading this book, I hope you will learn to appreciate who you are, rather than going to extremes to pour yourself into a mould in which you do not fit. In life, there is not one size, belief, or trend that fits all; that is the joy of being an individual—being you! After all, fitting your own mould is easier than fitting someone else's. Today I am happy being me, I hope you will be happy too!

· About the Author ·

When I was a teenager and in my twenties I had chronic acne, which hurt and stung when I used a flannel (washcloth) on my face. I did not know about natural solutions back then. I used antibiotic lotions from the doctor or dermatologist. Each time, I had high hopes the pills or lotions would work but the results rarely lasted. I was constantly disappointed. The cycle defined my life: disappointment and unhappiness. I felt immensely self-conscious and had very low self-esteem.

I covered up my acne with foundation which I now know contained synthetic chemical ingredients. Doctors prescribed endless pills and lotions and finally, I was advised by a dermatologist to take Roaccutane (known in the U.S.A. as Accutane), a synthetic drug. Thankfully, something made me think "Don't take it." I could not explain what it was but it was a strong feeling, so I listened. I so desperately wanted to have beautiful skin; I can remember crying myself to sleep many times as it seemed so hopeless. I am eternally grateful for that instinct not to take the Roaccutane. I did not go down the route of synthetic drugs but took dramatic action that was of an altogether more natural bias.

I left London for Australia, which, looking back, was a curious decision yet it was the turning point. Once there, I stayed in a Sydney hostel for a few weeks and then quite by chance got to share a flat with a vicar and his wife who were unbelievably kind to me. They welcomed me into their home and accepted me for who I am, something at the time I struggled to do myself.

Serendipity, faith, God moving in mysterious ways … call it what you will but my year in Australia taught me so much, mainly that today is what it is all about. Be grateful, be kind, live simply, take responsibility for your own health and above all be sure to laugh. I returned to the U.K. knowing there was hope.

The main change was my attitude but that is one of the most powerful things one can do! I began consciously to care for myself rather than expecting someone else to do it for me. I spent time in peace and quiet, listening to God as to where to go next. God says, "I will direct your steps", (Proverbs 3:6), and that He will "Send me in the right direction", (Psalm 23:1). Those words gave me great encouragement.

Throughout the book I will share stories from my life. As I am a Christian, they may involve reference to God. Having travelled a great deal in my life, I have noticed that most of us believe in a power, a spirit that is bigger than us, an entity we pray to, chat to, or whom we hope will be there if we find ourselves up the proverbial creek without a paddle. I have found that God IS there. I have been a Christian since 1998 and God has been my supporting guide ever since. I equally feel that you have to seek Him personally and, so, whilst it works for me, I know you are resourceful and competent enough to find what works for you.

Most fundamentally, my hope for you in reading this book is that you begin to like the woman you are and the woman you will be in twenty years' time. You are more radiant and precious than you might think.

Joanna Runciman
British Columbia
May 2013

PART ONE

. . .

Internal Care
of the
Radiant Woman

. . .

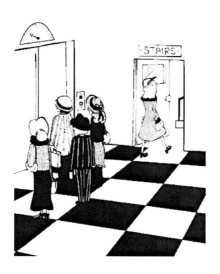

CHAPTER 1

. . .

Slowly, Slowly Change Your Life

. . .

If you are tempted to change everything all at once, be warned: a canoe does not change course quickly. It turns about gradually and that is what I urge you to do, too. Take your time; change the course of your canoe slowly. Before you say something negative like, "Oh, with my luck, I'll capsize", read on to discover why that negative thought is the first thing that has to go.

The key is to take gentle steps whilst going against the tide. If you want to be happy and healthy in today's society, that's what it's going to take: paddling against the tide. The common habits of eating low-nutrient junk food, going on crash diets and undertaking extreme skin care regimes are ones to leave behind. Unless that model is working for you, you will have to do things differently.

It is essential to do what best nourishes your body and soul. That may not be what your friends are doing or what you see in the media. Junk food and junk thinking can lead to unhappiness. Changing how you nourish your body and how you think about your body will benefit you and your loved ones.

So, first, you need to *claim* your radiance. No one can do that for you. Make this declaration with me right now to get started:

> *I wholeheartedly commit to being me. I, _____,*
> *am unique. I am going to stop comparing myself to airbrushed*
> *models and society-driven ideals. I am going to be me. I will be*
> *kind to myself each and every day, even if some days that means*
> *having a cup of tea and relaxing for ten minutes. I will honour my*
> *precious body. I accept I will do my best, which may be different*
> *on different days. Doing my best doesn't mean transforming into a*
> *super woman; it means merely* <u>being the best person possible—</u>
> <u>and being content with that.</u>

Signed:

_____

Signature

Sort the Positive from the Negative

In beginning the journey to become a more radiant you, it is important to understand the battle going on between positive and negative sides in your life. Modern life can grind you down—do you know that feeling?

I know I do. There is the busy-ness of life that overwhelms, the constant phone calls, emails, chores around the home, negative news stories, work commitments, family commitments and late at night worries— and that's just to name a few!

Many advertisements and media reports are designed to feed this feeling of pressure and, in some cases, the (insidious) goal is simply to persuade you to buy more 'stuff'. Think for a moment about how television shows portray modern life. How realistic are they? They certainly don't reflect my life!

Television shows range from the sublime to the ridiculous, from dramas portraying everything as perfect to the voyeuristic and extraordinarily bizarre 'reality' TV shows, where children dress up as beauty queens with fake nails and spray tans. None of these reflect real life for the majority of us. More often than not they are presenting us with unachievable goals that simply depress us.

In an increasingly disconnected world we might turn to social media rather than a cup of tea with a girlfriend to discuss the daily woes. Sherry Turkle, in her book *Alone Together,* writes that "technology promises to let us do anything from anywhere with anyone. But it also drains us as we try to do everything everywhere. We begin to feel overwhelmed and depleted by the lives technology makes possible."[1]

In sorting the positive from the negative, it is important to ask yourself where you are spending your time and how that suits you. For example, do you spend two hours on the Internet but sleep poorly and wish you had more time with family? Today many of us find time to be on the Internet yet complain we have no time, so perhaps it is just a case of reallocating where we spend our minutes and hours?

I must confess I dislike Facebook. It has led to some new connections, I must admit, but I am not entirely sure the whole business of updating the world about my day is healthy. The majority of posts are mere snippets of the real life being led, but can lead to a feeling of inadequacy when someone we know is (yet again) in Bali or sharing a menu from dinner at a top London or New York restaurant!

I also think it makes it too easy to take our family for granted. While we sit on social media sites, I know I am guilty of the dismissive, "Yes, I'll be there in a moment", as I do one last 'vital' search on the Internet. It is not vital; it is an addiction and one that I do not think has improved our relationships. I had to do some really firm talking to myself, as I was spending far too much time checking the computer and spending time with faces far away rather than enjoying those friends and family right here.

I know from my friends there is a lack of willingness to commit that has crept in to arranging dinner parties or meeting up. "I'll let you know", people say (*"unless something better comes up"*, we imply). Is this fear of missing out healthy? Is the last minute lifestyle serving us well?

I simply would rather interact on a face-to-face basis, perhaps as I like a cup of tea, but I also think it is more authentic and certainly more fun. You are welcome to say I am old-fashioned and I likely am but I think humans are wired to seek hugs, eye contact, smiles and compassion. I simply do not think social media gives that connection.

Dr. Amy Slater, from Flinders University in Australia, suggests that teenage girls using Facebook are unhappier with their body image and have more feelings of depression. According to Dr. Slater's studies, girls who spend less time on the Internet and more time doing their homework or reading have a more positive view of their bodies, less depressive feelings and a stronger sense of their own individual identity.[2] This is only one study but I imagine there will be scores more as new negative information about the ills caused by excessive computer time emerges.

Facebook has relentless adverts now and I often click spam or hide them, clicking the "offensive" button. I find an advert for weight loss offensive, especially as I do not need it! I find adverts about make up offensive, too. Yet, if I am feeling less than buoyant, I do notice the adverts and a little voice in my head says, "Oh, I wonder if that will help wrinkles?", or whatever the advert is touting. Once I've allowed that little niggling voice inside my head, it can be rather hard to shut it up.

What social media gives is yet another platform of boasting, comparisons and consumerism; it can eat away at beautiful women, who simply spend so much time wishing for things they do not have that they fail to notice what they do have. I know, as that is precisely what I used to do. These comparisons gave rise to a sense of not being good enough, which led me to think that purchasing a new top might fill the void. It did for a while, or so I thought. I really only started to find life more enjoyable when I accepted myself as I was rather than constantly comparing myself to something I wasn't. I claimed my radiance.

From Negative to Positive

When I recognised the positive and sorted out the negative influences on my life it made life simpler. It is less stressful knowing what is negative and not serving me well. That is half the battle—recognising what is beneficial in your life and what is not. You will spend less time worrying what others think as you will know what nourishes you and what drains you. This will not be the same for every person. I happen to love silence; others feel uneasy in silence. Thankfully we are all different.

Everything I have just said is far easier to write than do in real life but I have done it and I have proven it is possible. It is the only way to change this cycle. Changing and renewing your mind is the best way to start living in your radiance.

GIVE IT A GO

- Think about what you would like to change in your life—perhaps even write it in a journal. Often we limit our success by our thinking. So if you want to change something major, perhaps put that in your journal, too.
- Consider how much time you spend on social media and ask yourself how that is serving you. If you know you are addicted, why not have a day without turning the computer on?
- Jot down the positive influences in your life, jot down the negative too—are there any changes you could make?

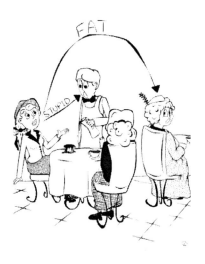

CHAPTER 2

. . .

Words Have Power, Lots of It!

. . .

Do not dismiss the serious power of your words. Have you ever said, "I hate my body", or "I never succeed at that"? I used to and funnily enough, I did. Yet, when I changed my thinking I reclaimed my life. It seems so simple written down but it really is life changing. I now say to myself, "I love my body" and it has definitely helped me accept myself the way I am.

Learning about the power of the words I speak all started when I was chatting with the vicar's wife (with whom I was living in Sydney, Australia back in 1999). She said, "Joanna, you have to make your thoughts captive to Jesus." What she meant was, don't let negative thoughts take hold. When you notice a negative thought, hand it over to the rubbish bin in the sky. A negative thought, if allowed to fester, can and will grow into more negative thoughts. Get rid of the negative thought as soon as you recognise it.

Quite rightly, you might be asking, "What on earth is the rubbish bin in the sky?" I was staying once with one of my oldest friends in London, telling him about something I had said to someone. He replied, "That should go to the rubbish bin in the sky." I am not sure what he actually said but that is what I heard. It's funny how sometimes we hear something that is not remotely what the person said; in this case, however, it was beneficial. I seized the imagery and have used it ever since.

If you have a thought that is negative towards yourself or someone else, unless it will help him or her (it's debatable if negative comments ever do), then put it in the 'rubbish bin in the sky.' Pack it up, send it off and get rid of it. This is a simplified view, perhaps, but adopting the practice might save a few tears and heartache.

If you work better with a visual aid, write down the negative comments, thoughts, or experiences on a piece of paper. Then, when you are ready, hand it over to the rubbish bin in the sky (or even just under your kitchen sink!). You can put it in the fire or shred it. However you dispose of it, it will free you to move on and say something more uplifting and positive.

Forgiving is also a very powerful act and whilst that is also infinitely easier to write than to do in practice, it does free you to move on. The inability to forgive is somewhat like a poison that harms you rather than the other person.

I was quite struck by something I once heard, which is that if we really understood how powerful our words were, we'd quite likely prefer silence to saying something negative. That thought changed my view of the words I spoke. I love silence now!

The idea of me loving silence is hysterical to those who knew me as a child and teenager. Arthur, an old-age pensioner who is a friend of our family, used to say to me, "Joanna, you're the only person I know that could talk a glass eye to sleep." I used to chat *a lot*, so let me encourage you to believe that people can change!

Replacing negative words with positive words is a habit and one that initially may feel impossible. With perseverance you can start to say more positive words than negative ones in a day. That isn't to say you won't ever say a negative word; well, at least I have not succeeded. If you do succeed, please write to me and let me know how you did it! My life is a constant lesson in learning. I am always learning that I can say nicer things!

Perhaps you are unsure if words are as important as I say they are? Think of a time when someone said you looked well or that dinner was delicious. How did you feel? Good, embarrassed, or happy, perhaps? Maybe your thinking overrode their kind comment and you automatically thought, "Well, the pie was a bit burnt and I should have done a salad rather than carrots", or, "The jeans I am wearing make me look fat; she doesn't really mean her compliment." See how negative thinking impacts kind words from others? Deflecting a kind word is a shame as words have power. Kind ones are particularly powerful.

Perhaps you think the words you say about yourself are not important. Let's see whether that really is the truth. Sit quietly and read these words (either aloud or in your head) and note how you feel in your body. Notice what sensation arises.

LOVE

JOY

KINDNESS

FAT

SOFT

BEAUTIFUL
STUPID
PEACE
UGLY
MORON
GORGEOUS
HEAVENLY

Imagine that every word you speak is a gift. Say only what helps, builds up and encourages. If you imagine your words wrapped up, perhaps you will be less inclined to wrap up a dog poo or razor blade; our words can be just as foul or dangerous. Our words can also be lovely, beautiful and kind. Think about how you talk to yourself and your family; are most of your words kind or unkind?

Gary Chapman, in his book *The Five Love Languages*,[3] talks about "words of affirmation" and how they can rekindle an ailing marriage once we know our partner's love language. Words are that powerful.

Unfortunately, I regularly fail at using them wisely even though I am aware of their power. I admit I am guilty of saying really deeply, unkind words to my husband but I also have said tender, kind, loving words to him. And as an aside, the kind words are far more likely to inspire him to empty the dishwasher! (Not that that's the only reason I speak kind words to him!)

Words can build up or they can harm, they can give life or end lives, they can encourage or exterminate. The verse below really helped me start to see what I could do in my life to change how I was thinking:

Summing it all up, friends, I'd say you'll do best by filling your minds and meditating on things true, noble, reputable, authentic, compelling, gracious—the best, not the worst; the beautiful, not the ugly; things to praise, not things to curse (Philippians 4:18).

It is not always easy to think positive thoughts more than negative ones, especially if you watch a lot of news, view extreme television or read negative newspaper stories. However, positive is going to encourage you and build you up, negative isn't.

I need this advice as much as anyone else. I used to be so negative and fed up with life. Yet my words were not speaking about a positive, powerful future. If there was a downside, I had an amazing propensity to see it! It was a default pattern, an addiction if you like, and it kept on going until I decided to change.

How you think is a habit, or a magnet, even. If you think lots of positive thoughts then, in turn, it is easier to think more positive thoughts. You can choose. Give it a go for an hour and see how you get on. Then progress to a day, a week, a month and so on. Please do not beat yourself up if you say something unkind about someone. We are human; by our very nature we are not perfect. Lighten up and do your best! But remember that talking about our joys is better than dwelling on the downsides of life. There will always be things we can moan about (the world is not perfect) but I do not have to talk about the negatives of life. I can choose to use uplifting words and encourage myself and others with the powerful words I speak.

I particularly like the four agreements outlined in the book of the same name, *The Four Agreements*, by Don Miguel Ruiz. He also says taking things personally is pointless and does no good. I think he has a point! All four of the agreements are life changing. They free you to make and keep life a lot more simple.

The four agreements are:

1. **"Don't take things personally."**
2. **"Do your best."**
3. **"Be impeccable with your words."** (Say what you mean and speak the truth.)
4. **"Don't make assumptions."**[4]

Also remember that there is no one else in the world today who can be you. Celebrate knowing who you are, who you have been called to be—that is *you*! So whatever lies you have believed about not being good enough, please be assured that you are a treasure. What will you believe, words spoken in anger or your Creator's truth? Perhaps you think, "Yes, Joanna, that applies to others but not to me." Please do not be deceived; that is a lie. You are marvelously made! *"Body and soul, I am marvelously made"* (*Psalm 139:14*)!

Be you, be young, be old, be free, be messy, be tidy, be funny, but above all else...say good things about yourself and be YOU!

Love the Life You Live Now

I wonder how many hours you have spent dreaming of a different life? All this time wanting perhaps slimmer thighs, clearer skin, nicer toes, softer hair, wrinkle-free skin, longer nails, to be richer, to have a nicer house—when life is out there for you to grab. I must have wasted months of my life looking in magazines or at television programmes hoping miraculously to change my life. I do regret it. To this day I have no idea HOW I thought that would happen without changing my thinking and attitudes! Please don't *you* waste a moment more.

Today is where we are, tomorrow has not arrived and yesterday has gone. I can choose how I feel about what is happening around me in this moment.

It is refreshing to make a conscious decision to release resistance and start choosing to feel happy in all things. Think of two people who have the same illness whose journeys and attitudes are so different: they simply choose to look at life differently. And of course, they get different results.

I made a powerful decision to let go, to relax about my life. I made a simple choice to do my best. I began to fulfill my life's purpose and be the woman I was designed to be. I hope you can do that, too. But first let me clarify. Accepting who I am does not mean I never set goals or intentions; I do—lots of them! But I would not aim for unachievable goals and expect them to happen without work.

In the past, by wasting so much of my energy on futile wishes, I did not have time left to focus on the things that did matter. Having arrived at a place where I am happy being me, I am now able to conserve energy and use that to write a book, improve my skiing, grow, teach Nia, cook more for my family and write another book.

It is life changing living in the present rather than wishing your life away with, "I'll be happy when…" thoughts. I used to think like that and it did me little good. I now visit an art gallery, go to a comedy show, brush my teeth with the opposite hand, and stand on one leg washing up. Why not? It challenges my brain and keeps life interesting. Who says childlike curiosity has to stop when we get to 20 or 30? Branch out and be brave!

My grandmother will often go to the theatre to see a play when it opens just because she thinks it sounds good. Despite her age, she is unafraid of doing something she has not done before. I asked her about it and she said, "Well darling, you just have to get on and do things or you'll sit at home lonely." How wise she is.

I realise I spent much of my life thinking, "Oh, maybe there is something better going on" and then never going to anything. In recent years I have been much happier to commit to going to a film, restaurant, or play without worrying if something better will come along. If it does, so be it. But in my 38 years free concert tickets have not landed on my desk—at least not yet!

The fear of missing out is quite common, as is the anxiety of not knowing what to do. As 'friends' share their life on social media sites, the lack of commitment and subsequent empty feeling that we are missing out grows. It is insidious, and I find organising events very difficult as the 'let's text nearer the time' often means nothing happens .

FOMO (or "fear of missing out") it is called and I think modern communications and technology are a major reason why we see so much of it. I find it very annoying that people rarely commit these days. The ease with which a text message (changing plans) can be sent allows the issue to perpetuate.

I have been called a dinosaur before so I do not take offence if you think I am somewhat peculiar. What I have learnt is that by waiting for something better to happen, nothing happens and I can end up spending endless time that blends into days of "what-did-I-do-other-than-work".

So go to the art galley, see that film, learn to sew, go to that sporting event—or you may find that your life is a series of "could have been" moments.

GIVE IT A GO

- For a week, track (without judgment) how you talk about yourself and your life. Write down the words in a journal if you like, or just observe yourself. Be conscious and notice whether the first words that come to mind on waking are kind or condemning.

- Become aware of how you react to a compliment; do you simply say, "Thank you" and accept it? Or do you deflect it with a "What, this old coat? Oh I have had it for ages!" From now on, when someone pays you a compliment, simply pause, look into his or her eyes and say, "Thank you." It is far more powerful. So enjoy hearing and sharing positive words.

- A radiant woman knows the power of her words and uses them wisely, never to manipulate but to give joy. You can choose to think uplifting thoughts rather than critical ones. You can speak positive words rather than negative ones and you can learn to love the life you're living now instead of longing for one you may never see.

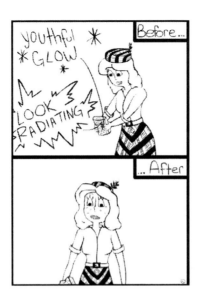

CHAPTER 3

. . .

Advertising's Little Secret

. . .

"You can fool all the people all the time
if the advertising is right and the budget is big enough".
Joseph E. Levine

Adverts are not for your benefit. Learn what is harming you through them so that you can choose radiance.

Much on television these days is not realistic but the adverts are especially unreal. Have you really watched them? Some of my girlfriends do not have a TV (they are very wise!); we still do but I am very careful what I watch. We record most things and fast forward adverts!

When I was at university I studied consumer psychology for a semester (I found it fascinating) and what I learnt was that most of the adverts on television and in magazines are designed to make you feel inadequate in order to sell you more stuff. They play on your insecurities (don't worry, we all have a few!) and, by playing on your vulnerability, they captivate you and make you willing to buy what they are selling.

In order to know what you are up against, sit down one day and pretend you are an analyser of adverts. Look at them through beginner's eyes. Look critically at the advert and you will see what is really happening. Ask yourself, is it playing on a weakness someone might have, an emotional point? Are they using insidious tactics? Notice how many adverts are implying, not so subtly, that you are:

too fat

too small

too old

too young

not sexy enough

too wrinkly

too tired

in need of a (sexy) man

too unambitious

too poor

wearing the wrong perfume

sporting the wrong watch

driving the wrong car

in the wrong job

under the wrong health care package

under-insured

too lazy

not pale enough

not brown enough
using an out of date mobile phone or computer
not looking after your children properly
being too protective

... and on and on the subliminal messages continue; essentially saying you are not complete unless you buy this product, this service, buy into this lifestyle, this group or way of thinking. Advertisements are designed to sell things and make money. They are not necessarily beneficial for your well-being.

Many adverts are outright negative messages. This is only so the product they are selling fills the gap. For example, if you are too fat, use this food to fill the gap. If you are too old, this cream will make you look younger in only 'this many days'. Read the small print on the television, it usually says 'tested on 100 women of whom 30 thought they might look better'!

The Cons of Advertising

"Advertising has these people chasing cars and clothes they don't need.
Generations have been working in jobs they hate,
just so they can buy what they don't really need."
Chuck Palahniuk, *Fight Club*

How right he is!
For years I bought products based on what the sales assistant said. Let me be clear, I am not blaming them; they have a job to do and I genuinely believe and know from personal experience they are not aware of the synthetic chemicals in much of skin care today. However, I bought products from them that I did not need—often fabulously expensive products bearing outrageous claims. As I was in a vulnerable position,

wanting to get rid of my acne, I just paid up. I wanted to look like the beautiful pictures on the department store stand; I wanted clear skin, a fresh-looking countenance and radiance.

Thankfully, I now have it but I did not get it by using much of what you can buy for $100 in glossy boxes. You get the glossy box, but what else? Advertisements for skin care are particularly misleading; they say one thing on the jazzy packaging—claims of wrinkles diminished, corrected skin blemishes, lines filled and smoothed. However, the ingredients say something entirely different: bio-accumulative substances and endocrine disruptors.

I know this having spent years reading about the subject. It upsets me that unless you are a label sleuth you are likely to be buying creams that contain potentially harmful ingredients. It still staggers me that some of the adverts are allowed on television, as they really imply that the little tub of cream is going to pretty much do a full facial makeover!

It's Just Fashion, Darling!

Fast forward from skin care to clothing. Who chooses what shoes you buy? Seriously? Having shoes is one thing but constantly wanting new ones, so that it overtakes your thinking, is unhealthy. My mother says with a smile, "Good teeth, happy face and clean nails are all you need—and some clothes might be good, too."

On a recent trip to the U.S.A., someone stole my raincoat. It was a nice coat; it fitted well, was stylish and I was regularly complimented on it. I now have to wear my old coat from the 1990s; it is not trendy and I do not get compliments. However, it is still a very waterproof jacket that keeps me warm and dry despite being somewhat retro. So why should that concern me?

I am not the height of fashion but I know what style I like: classic, English and some say quirky. And whilst I do not buy the latest designer clothes, I do like to smarten up my wardrobe now and again. The stolen raincoat was an uncomfortable reminder that I was more affected by fashion trends than I'd like to admit. None of us should believe themselves less of a person when sporting last year's clothes or shoes. Feeling so conscious of it shows the extent to which we are all victims of fashion at some time or other.

Perhaps you can relate to being conscious of what you are wearing? I think it is important to notice if you are overly anxious about what you wear. It is too easy to outsource your choices to magazines, adverts on TV and shop windows. I look at much of fashion today and think, "Oh boy, the emperor's new clothes designer was called in for that one!" and I walk on. Other times I think I'll just try on those skinny jeans. What ensues is a hilarious battle between my calves and a pair of jeans that were designed for a doll and not my happy thirties body! I end up handing back the jeans to the assistant (who looks young enough to be my daughter) and think to myself, "Boot cut jeans are classic; I'll stick with them!"

The Air Brush: Enemy of Women Everywhere

Many advertisements are nothing short of modern day highway robbery—just without the man with a cape and a flintlock pistol! You voluntarily buy magazines with glossy airbrushed pictures and pay to make yourself feel *like* rubbish. When you are feeling dissatisfied, unhappy, vulnerable or lonely, that is the perfect time for the adverts to make you feel like you want to buy a fabulously expensive face cream, which may or may not work.

I used to buy magazines, at least three glossy magazines each month. With my chronic acne I struggled, as each model looked utterly beautiful with flawless, clear, youthful skin. When I looked in the mirror all I saw was imperfection. Yes, I had acne but HOW SILLY of me; there was perfection there… under construction. I just didn't see it. That is not me being arrogant but simply claiming my radiance.

I am beautiful; I have to believe it first. You are beautiful and you have to believe it, too. Stop comparing yourself! This is the number one mistake smart women make that keeps them feeling insignificant and unhappy. Truly embracing who you are is the key to radiant happiness. Comparing yourself to others does little for your self-esteem or long-term happiness. When you accept yourself as you are, the pressure is off to conform to the airbrushed images in magazines. It really is a great relief.

Many images are tweaked and enhanced so much. If you compare a magazine picture to those pictures of you, taken with your own camera, it is recipe for feeling low and inadequate. I used to compare myself constantly; it made me utterly miserable. Back in the '90s I had no idea that magazines were airbrushed and so I just thought I was not as good as the stunning picture of Christy Turlington or Cindy Crawford.

My cousin is very pretty, tall (she is nearly six feet) and she is a model. Yet when I see her in a magazine she somehow looks different from when I see her at Granny's house for lunch. That is not to say she is not very striking and pretty (she is both) but if they airbrush very pretty models then I think we are foolish to think that models look like they do in the magazines in real life!

That's why comparing yourself to women in magazines is a recipe for unhappiness. That isn't to say there are not some very beautiful people in the world but the vast majority of us are not going to grace the cover of a magazine. That is okay and doesn't make us any less valued than those women who do. It is refreshing to embrace being you as there is no pressure to look thin, fat, tall, short, brown, young or old since you are you; unique.

Many women today seem to be on a diet and their obsession with calories must be grueling. I recently put on ten pounds; I only know as I weighed myself at the spa and I hadn't been for about six months. Last time I weighed myself I was ten pounds lighter! I don't weigh myself normally. I just know that my jeans are either fitting or a bit snug, as they currently are.

I know why I have put on weight, though. I had the flu and was in bed for a week. Then I have been writing my book and so I have not been taking as much exercise. I am not feeling bad or unhappy. I simply know that I have to eat a little bit less at supper and get a brisk walk every day. I am not suddenly going to eat lettuce leaves; I will see how my jeans fit and monitor it.

Aside from the fact that many magazine pictures are airbrushed, there are women literally starving themselves in order to fit an image they think is attractive. Yet a tummy is not a bad thing. I have one, don't you? So why are flat stomachs so sought after? I used to have one but I also had chronic digestive issues. Now I am happy to wear a dress and see my tummy. I don't feel fat; I just know that there is less tension there. Constantly pulling in your tummy is so tiring, or is it just me who thinks this?

Eating Well

Whilst eating good food and taking exercise is important, so is finding balance and being happy with the body you have today. Perhaps we need more body acceptance and less of the 'I'll be happen when I've lost ten pounds'. I must admit I have got much more accepting of my body and I do not look like I am 20 any more, but that is totally okay.

Real radiance, I think, is a softness, a glow and a calmness—not a "go-go-go foot on the brake and accelerator body". Surely peaceful radiance comes from eating nourishing food and not stressing your body through denial.

If you want your body to serve you well and look well, you must feed it regularly and properly. We'll talk more about that later in an upcoming chapter. It's important!

GIVE IT A GO

- Next time you are looking at magazines or billboards, ask yourself, "Am I comparing myself?" When clothes shopping and something doesn't fit, do you start with the self-berating or are you okay with it? Just notice, no judgement.
- Are you choosing a style and colours that you really enjoy and feel happy wearing or are you buying something simply as it is "in fashion?"
- Are you aiming at a target weight based on a desire to look a certain way?
- Could you change your focus and accept yourself, as you are, today?

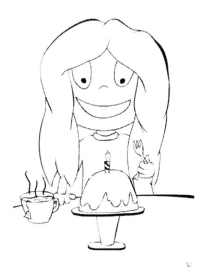

CHAPTER 4

. . .

Gratitude and Living NOW

. . .

What are you grateful for today?

If nothing comes to mind (or very little), then you are likely living, as I did for years, with that thought of "I'll be happy when... (fill in the blank)". The reality of life is if we let our circumstances dictate how we feel, it is not a good recipe for joy.

I used to think that stuff—new shoes, smart car, nice house and beautiful clothes—would make me happy. Those are all very nice but they do not make me happy. My brain makes me happy. Daniel Gilbert, author of *Stumbling into Happiness*, talks about how happiness can be synthesized. Yet despite our ability to synthesize happiness, we also believe that happiness has to be found. Gilbert says the freedom to choose is the enemy of synthetic happiness; i.e. if we had no choice but one pair of shoes, we would find ourselves synthesizing that we were happy with those shoes. It is just the way our clever brains work.[5]

In his book *Thanks!*, Robert A. Emmons shares how powerful it is to want what we have rather than wanting what we do not have. Gratitude is finding things in your life for which you are thankful, things that make you happy. Reading this book motivated me to start saying, "I am happy because......(fill in the blank)" and start a gratitude journal. The amazing thing about a journal of gratitude is that when you say, "I am happy or grateful for .... (something)", you will invariably find another thing you are grateful for and so it snowballs into a lot of things about which you are happy. Giving thanks is contagious when we genuinely mean it.

Gratitude (like our words) is very powerful—addictive even (in a good way). By thinking of things for which you are grateful, you often notice even more! Just like a smile can make you feel better when you are annoyed, gratitude can help you gain perspective when things are not going your way.

Gratitude is also thought to improve sleep. Studies at Manchester University, England, concluded "Gratitude predicted greater subjective sleep quality and sleep duration."[6] Whilst subjective, it may still be worth thinking of things you are grateful for before going to bed, especially if you are struggling to sleep. Robert A Emmons says, "If you want to sleep more soundly, count blessings, not sheep."[7]

My husband was once in a serious skiing accident. He needed a major operation and whilst it was scary and I cried a lot, I was eternally grateful it was only his leg that was injured. I kept saying, *"Thank you."* I am so grateful we were blessed with a great surgeon who operated on him quickly and did an excellent job. *"Thank you"* that we had savings to rely on when he could not work and the insurance company did everything they could to not help us. "*Thank you*" that I could still find things to be smiling about even when he was in much pain. I could have been angry that he was hurt; I went through that emotion too, but in the main I was just grateful he was safe and we lived in a country where good medical treatment was available.

Ask yourself: what are you grateful for? It may, initially, just be something like a glass of fresh water or a comfy bed and a hot cup of tea. But after a while you'll be surprised how much you can notice and how that allows you the opportunity to notice more. It is "like finding like" in a way and that is really fun, as it is contagious. I may be feeling grateful one day and will say in a bus queue, "Oh, look at the beautiful clouds." Someone else will notice and agree; they then smile and so it goes on. A smile is sometimes the most powerful gift (and expression of your inner gratitude) that you can give someone. It might be the only smile they see all day.

Don't Let "Lack" Steal Your Joy

Forgive me for saying this but one of the worst things about North American and British culture is the insidious "lack" disease: the desire to have more and more stuff—more clothes, a bigger TV, a new car, more shoes and more DVDs—you name it. Surely wanting more simply creates unhappiness and a "lack mentality"?

How do you recognize a "lack mentality" in yourself? You have a general feeling of unhappiness, you feel hard done by and you want more from life. You always have something you want to buy and having bought something you know what you want to buy next. You are annoyed at how other people behave and make you feel. A "lack mentality" is quite like a victim mentality. It is very common in the modern world and even though many of us are so abundantly blessed, we still want more.

Perhaps you have a good job and are well paid but you still feel empty, unhappy and hungry for more. You have great clothes but don't like any of them. You think "I'll be happy when I have that new handbag" (or it could be a new lawnmower but you get the idea!).

The "lack mentality" is a way of thinking and can be stopped. I know as I used to be unhappy and often wanting more and blaming everyone around me and yet it was simply my attitude to life. I wanted more yet it wasn't until I stopped and realised how grateful I was that I came to love what I had and now I rarely want more.

You can reduce the sense of lack and create more gratitude in your life by thanking others and being grateful for their part in your life. Thank the person on the cash register at the supermarket; look her in the eye and say, "Thank you." See what happens. Usually the response will be one of (returned) gratitude, which feels good for them and you. Being grateful helps bring perspective and radiance to your life.

Body Gratitude

I've learnt to express my radiance by being grateful for my own body. This is also often a focus in a Nia 5 Stages class, which consists of five movements based on the developmental stages of human development: embryonic, creeping, crawling, standing and walking. Moving the body with gratitude is powerful.

Debbie Rosas, co-creator of Nia, says "The first step is to notice, tune in to what you sense in your body; for example, whilst sitting reading, say 'I notice my hands.' Then move them, wiggle your fingers, scrunch them up and open them. Then tune in and notice if they feel different; say, 'Thank you, body; I sense my hands are warmer. Thank you, body; I sense the tips of my fingers.'"

Consciously loving and accepting myself started when I did my Nia White Belt. I had never taken a Nia class before but soon after starting the training I realised that moving, dancing and martial arts were a way to be strong, feminine and to laugh more. It really has made a great difference in my life.

A brief word about Nia: Nia is an expressive movement and life-style practice that is based on the joy of movement. It is practised in bare feet. Being fun, Nia is easier to keep doing than many exercise regimes; it is far more inviting than thrashing myself on a treadmill. I vividly remember my first Nia class in 2005. I said to the teacher, "I hate my feet." She replied, "Well, kick off your shoes, dance and see how you get on." Seven years later, I have just completed my Nia Brown Belt and I love my feet; they keep me dancing on the earth and are strong and allow me to walk to where I am going.

Learn to love yourself! It is possible. Showing myself love may just be going for a walk in the sunshine (or rain), moisturising my nails, making a cup of tea and settling down with a good book or putting on a favourite song and dancing for a few minutes. I find I can now tap into the sensation of JOY wherever I am—cooking, cleaning the basin, driving or gardening. Noticing the sensation of joy allows me to let time stand still. I have found that mindfully taking time to do an activity allows me to enjoy it wholeheartedly without distractions. I don't think that is the norm today.

Living Forward or Living NOW?

I live in a place where, come winter, I can enjoy superb skiing nearby. Curiously, throughout the beautiful hot summer people say to me, "So, are you looking forward to winter?" This question puzzles me greatly as I have been asked it so many times. Snow will not fall for months, so I am curious as to why someone would be looking forward to winter when it will be freezing cold (as low as -20C/ -4F). It isn't that I do not like winter but I enjoy it *when it arrives*; I don't look forward to it. I have not been looking forward or looking back, I simply enjoy today.

I think this is paramount in radiant living, being fully in today, this moment, rather than looking back or way into the future. Being in the moment, without distractions, might be uncommon today as many are preoccupied with their mobile phones at dinner, whilst meeting friends for a drink, or even at business meetings. This disconnection might now be socially acceptable (not in my house though, so remember that!) but I just wonder what it is hiding. Our insecurities? Our fears? It certainly has become a habit, this living elsewhere rather than here in the present.

I wonder how many times you live forward, looking forward to things rather than being fully present in today? I often hear, "I'm bored", uttered by adults and teenagers alike. Yet if I am fully present boredom flees. Right now, I see the bright morning sunshine beaming on the tree outside my office, and the bold chickadee hopping along the sunlit branch. You get the idea. Boredom for many of us is an attitude of mind. Tune in to living now and you may start to notice just how incredible the world around you is!

Contentment in Your Own Space

Do you want to know how to free up your thinking and enjoy having enough today? Try getting rid of some stuff.

Clutter is overwhelming. In North America and parts of Europe many of us are buying more stuff than we need, not just a little bit more than we need but a LOT more! How much do you really *need*? It is likely a lot less than you think you need.

I have felt more peace and joy since I have been conscious of "stuff" and realised there is more space in my life for joy when I have less stuff around. It is liberating. I now ask of all my purchases, "Is this really going to make me happy or am I just being greedy?" I also wait a few days before buying something and very often I realise I did not really want it anyway.

To want more and more—never feeling satisfied—is *exhausting*. It also means we are never able to just "be" as our thoughts are always far off, wanting. To be fair, society and modern business have designed it that way to make us buy more.

Things don't last like they used to, have you noticed? Think how many times you've heard this said in the shops: "Actually, we can't even repair them now", or, "They design them to break", or "You could repair it but it'll cost you more than a new one", or, "They don't even make spare parts; we can't get them." This baffles me as we live in a world where we need to be mindful of our consumerism, in order to lessen our impact on the planet, not create more waste!

More clothes, more food (think how food has changed over the years—more food in packaging), more phones, more DVDs, more cars, more technology and more stuff... AGGHH!

You do not need to buy into the more-clutter habit. It is possible to enjoy life without potentially over-extending yourself keeping up with the latest trends. Last year, for Christmas, our family did not give presents for the sake of presents, we only gave things we knew the other person would use, eat, wear, or really wanted. Mum made me a beautifully warm winter nightie, my sister gave me a retro woollen jumper (sweater) and Dad gave me some tea bags, a garden tarpaulin for collecting all the leaves and a pencil. You might think that sounds like a boring Christmas? No way! The pencil is really cool, with animals on it, the tea is a brand of tea I can't get in Canada and I am grateful for all these presents - as they are all things I love and will use. I think of Dad each time I use the pencil and I am wearing the jumper my sister gave me today!

Free Yourself (from Entitlement)

Modern advertising, as I have said, would have you believe that creams, potions, diets and new clothes are what you need in order to look and feel radiant, complete and happy. However, that is not true. In contrast, some of the happiest people I have met live in frugal circumstances, wear second hand clothes and have very, very few material possessions.

If you have a television and spare clothes, then you are materially richer than some people I have met in Africa who are genuinely happy.

The curious thing is that they *could* be unhappy: they could complain that their wild animals are being poached; their children get malaria and die and they have daily struggles with reliable sources of clean water. Despite all this they decide to choose happiness. Generally speaking, I find they choose to look at life with a spirit of joy.

You have that choice, too. Will you take it?

GIVE IT A GO

- Each morning before you get out of bed, tune in. Notice how your toes feel; your eyes feel as they look about the bedroom; notice what you can see. Sense: is your tongue relaxed or pressed on the roof of your mouth? As you wash your face, notice the warm water on your skin. Enjoy it, without guilt! Be grateful for it.

- Remember: Body awareness and subsequent body gratitude are powerful.

- Set an intention for the day that you will stop each hour and thank a part of your body that you have just used. For example, after making a cup of tea say, "Thank you, hands, for your precise grip on the kettle." It may feel strange but what you are doing is bringing positive thoughts into the forefront of your awareness. I bet you'll find yourself smiling more!

- Choose happiness in a situation where you may not have done so in the past.

- Can you simplify things?

- Can you clear out some clutter?

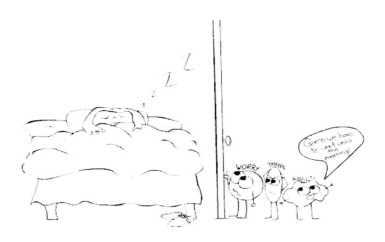

CHAPTER 5

. . .

Sleep

. . .

Why have I included an entire chapter on sleep? Sleep is important, that is why. If you are running on empty all the time from late nights, parties, worries and sleep deprivation, chances are your skin will not glow and you will struggle to feel vibrant during your day. When you sleep well, you feel better, think more clearly and look infinitely more radiant! "Sleeping is not time wasting."[8]

Sadly, we do not all get the sleep we need. I was astonished to read on a *New York Times* blog that in 2011 Americans filed nearly 60 million prescriptions for sleeping pills. About one in every seven

Canadians "(has) problems going to sleep or staying asleep and thus are considered to have insomnia."[9] In the UK, "10 million prescriptions for sleeping pills (hypnotics) are written annually in England alone."[10]

Lack of sleep is a modern epidemic but whilst many of us are concerned with eating well and exercising somehow sleep gets missed. Yet it is restorative and calming, since "a good night's sleep can really help a moody person decrease their anxiety. You get more emotional stability with good sleep."[11]

I have a friend who regularly says, "I pulled another all-nighter, just working crazy-long hours at the moment. I did an 18-hour day yesterday." I don't think sleep is negotiable or simply an area we can ignore in favour of getting more work done. Whilst in the short-term we may tick things off our to-do list, what are the long-term effects?

There are also rather more serious consequences from constant sleep deprivation, such as anxiety and depression, impairment of memory and concentration, poor decision making, increased irritability and risk taking, impaired immune response, increased risk of metabolic disorders and diabetes and increased risk of some cancers.[12] Sleep is vital, important and necessary!

There are many theories as to why we sleep, including cellular restoration, energy conservation, consolidation of memory and learning.[13] I can vouch for the consolidation of memory and learning; whilst writing this book, the overwhelming temptation, when very "into" a subject or chapter at 7:00 p.m., was to keep going late into the night. Yet, I refrained. I know the value of sleep and actually have been far more productive by turning off the computer, having supper, chatting, having a hot bath, sleeping and waking up refreshed.

Quality of sleep is also important. Many of us complain of feeling tired but are we creating conditions conducive to a good night's sleep? Often not! Many check their emails on a computer or mobile phone just before bed or perhaps even bring their hand held tablet to bed. What about that work email that actually makes you angry; surely that can wait until the morning? What happens in all these scenarios is that the body gets sleep but not the high quality sleep that it needs.

As I mentioned earlier, I recently had flu—the first time in at least 15 years that I had to go to bed for more than a day! Yet, I found that the rest, recuperation and prolonged times of sleep brought me immense clarity. By not being able to get up and busy myself, I had to tune in to the present moment and allow life to happen rather than making it happen. It was hugely refreshing.

Busy is a much over-used word; "I'm too busy", "I can't, I'm too busy", "I'd love to but I'm too busy". I recognise saying those phrases, often. Recently, with writing my book, I have had to be disciplined to take time for myself; schedule rest, a day off, meet a girl friend for lunch and stop allowing work distractions to dominate. I was doing too much racing here and there. There will always be work to do; the key is to know when to take time off.

Being busy is a distraction and I am sure that doing nothing, resting and sleeping are all good cures for modern life. I am not suggesting we all do nothing but sleep, however, sometimes stopping long *enough* to "be" can be very powerful.

I wonder if the vast lack of sleep in our society is a factor in why so many are angry, irrational, frustrated or sad and suffer from rage whilst simply waiting in the queue at the post office. Trust me, in the run up to Christmas, I saw it a lot! People huffing and puffing, swearing and carrying on but none of that made the queue move any faster!

I don't think sleep is a negotiable part of life, although clearly many feel it is, sacrificing sleep for a quick check of their social media updates. Can you relate? The computer and phone both have off buttons, as far as I know! (Well, mine do and I use them, daily.)

It is time to alter our habits?

Tips for Better Sleep

I am always amazed by the adverts for sleeping pills on the television. My mother and father were staying with us a few years ago, my father was watching an American channel (sport most likely) and the story went like this (I'm paraphrasing the advert): 'Try this sleeping pill and ask your doctor if it is right for you', (cut to musical piece) followed by an alarming list of potential side effects including 'may cause nausea and erectile dysfunction.' My father promptly replied "Crikey! You'd prefer a sleepless night over that lot!" It was really funny but I am under no illusion that insomnia isn't. Even so, I would not want to take a pill that has such alarming potential side effects, certainly not when alternative solutions exist.

Few cultures do much to promote the value of sleep and often the only "solution" is medication. The Canadian sleeping pill market is growing and according to market research firm IMS Brogan the number of sedative prescriptions increased from 16.4 million in 2006 to more than 20 million in 2011.[14]

Some say lack of sleep can be caused by stress yet the tricky thing is that lack of sleep causes more stress and anxiety. (It's a bit like the age-old question of what came first, the chicken or the egg?) The secret is to get into a habit of prioritising sleep, be disciplined, consciously relax and wind down earlier than you want to go to bed. As with any habit you will likely fight it when you first start. Perhaps you think you do unwind, by watching television—but watching a James Bond film before bed is unlikely to relax you!

Here are some ideas that can help you unwind and sleep more soundly:

1. Guard your mind.

Your mind is susceptible to what it sees. That is why watching TV shows containing disturbing content before bed is unwise (well, it's probably not great any time of day but definitely worse just before bedtime!). Unwinding before bed is vital if you want your body to feel relaxed and ready to sleep. Why not play a game (I always get beaten at Scrabble!), crochet or read a book rather than sitting in front of the computer or television, which can actually *over*stimulate the body? Some experts say we should avoid having a television in the bedroom altogether, I agree wholeheartedly!

2. Rest your brain.

Silence is healing. Many go to retreats to rest and recuperate with no talking for days, so why not have some quiet time before bed?

Do your best to create a positive atmosphere. Spend a moment recalling things you are grateful for from your day (as we spoke about in the last chapter). It can relax the body and calm the mind. Gratitude is a positive tool to master and is thought to assist with sleep.[15]

3. Take a bath

A warm to hot bath can raise the body temperature and that is thought to assist with inducing sleep. I find I sleep really well after a bath! You may also want to add essential oils to your bath to aid relaxation. I use lavender oil, which is thought to help relax the mind, ease insomnia and lessen anxiety. You can also use a drop on the pillow to calm your mind. Perhaps it is placebo or perhaps not.[16] I love chamomile too!

4. Exercise regularly

Getting adequate exercise during the day can help you sleep better at night. A recent study reported by NBC News said that women who exercised (at least 45 minutes of moderate walking or riding a stationary bike) five days a week averaged 70 percent better sleep than women who didn't![17] (The caveat was that it was morning exercise that encouraged better sleep. Those who exercised at night ended up being more wakeful.) Morning exercise also ensures you get exposed to brighter sunlight, which is an important part of a healthy sleep cycle.

5. Create a sleep-friendly environment

- Get up and go to bed at the same time each day if possible.
- Turn your mobile phone(s) off at night. (If you use your mobile phone as an alarm clock, then for $10 or so you can buy a battery operated normal alarm clock, not one with lit up numbers but an old fashioned alarm clock.)
- Make sure your room is tranquil and uncluttered. (Your bedroom is a place for sleep, sex, maybe reading a book—but not paying bills online or dealing with clutter. The less mess the better.)
- Avoid having a television in your bedroom.
- Do not drink lots of water before bed, as that can disrupt your sleep when you need to pee.
- Sleep in a totally darkened room that is cool in temperature, roughly 16 to 18C (62 to 66F). Open a window to get fresh air; if you feel cold in bed snuggle up with a hot water bottle, bed socks, or an extra woollen blanket.

I want to make a specific comment about using the computer in bed, which seems like an easy and innocuous practice but really isn't. Sara Thomée and her research colleagues at the University of Gothenburg's Sahlgrenska Academy in Sweden found that "regularly using a computer late at night is associated not only with sleep disorders but also with stress and depressive symptoms in both men and women." [18]

Shutting the computer down two hours before bedtime can allow your body to start to wind down in order to rest when you do fall asleep. The bright light from the computer screen may well over-stimulate you, making you feel more alert.[19] Turning your computer off before bed may seem a tough challenge but it is possible and I can assure you that your sleep will be greatly enhanced. The nights that I manage to wind down long before bed and rest, I sleep deeply and wake feeling refreshed. The very occasional times I think, "Ooh, I will read the British paper before bed" on my iPad®, I find my brain is whirring long after I stop reading. I still sleep but wake wanting more sleep.

If you have a computer then there is a free programme called F.lux[20], which actually sets your time zone and when dusk falls the light on your computer gets much dimmer. I use it and whilst I am not on the computer very late, I find it really stops the overstimulation from a bright screen.

I was very fortunate to have a long telephone conversation with Professor Russell Foster of Oxford University on the subject of sleep. I concluded that sleep is the missing link in our modern day health issues and currently we have an epidemic of sleep deprivation. Professor Foster says it is particularly noticeable among Britain's teenagers. He has been studying the effect of light on our sleep and we spend so much time indoors that this is essentially disrupting our circadian clock.

We have to get sunshine on our eyes and face in order to set our internal clock. Those living in cities are thought to get a form of jet-lag from lack of available sunlight on a regular basis, yet those in the coun-tryside appear to get more natural light.[21]

We agreed that there needs to be more teaching of the *value* of sleep in schools, colleges and workplaces so we start to turn around the "go-go-go sleep is for wimps lifestyle" and actually get good qual-ity sleep on a regular basis.

'Earthing' as a Sleep Aid

Being "earthed" is another increasingly popular way of perhaps assisting poor sleep. Think how good it feels to walk barefoot on the grass or beach. That calm feeling can be recreated by sleeping on earthed bed sheets, according to Clint Ober in his book, *Earthing*.[22] John Gray (author of *Men are from Mars, Women are from Venus*) writes, "The concept of earthing resonates deeply with me. I have, in fact, done something similar since 1995 when I was in India … It was recommended to me that for the best results in my practice I should sleep and meditate on deerskin, and the deerskin should be on the ground … (that) there was energy from above that comes to the earth and then comes to you if you stay connected to the earth."[23]

When did you last kick off your shoes? We thrive when connected to the earth. Children very often will take their shoes off and blissfully run about the garden. Even in winter I have seen children hurtling about in bare feet, giggling away with delight. We can learn from their childlike instincts. I love walking on the grass barefoot or lying down reading a book.

Being connected to the earth is how we always used to live before concrete roads, multi-level tower blocks and plastic soled shoes. Emerging scientific research supports the concept that the earth's electrons induce multiple physiological changes of clinical significance, including reduced pain and better sleep.[24] It is thought that we may discharge energy by walking barefoot or sitting on the ground. By constantly wearing shoes, we are losing the ability to ground our body as we would naturally do wearing leather soled shoes rather than plastic or rubber.

As much as it seems I am suggesting the old fashioned ways are the best, I think we can have the best of both worlds. The benefits of a modern world mean that I can pick up the phone and chat to my

Mother, in England, for two cents a minute from North America whilst accessing her wisdom from years past.

I feel we can slow down a bit; kick off our shoes and breathe out the day's worries, have a hot bath and sink into bed for a restful night's sleep. Modern living and ancient wisdom provide the perfect balance.

GIVE IT A GO

- For a week (or longer if you are willing), turn your computer off straight after dinner in the evening. Enjoy an activity that is not looking at a lit screen; perhaps prepare some food for the next day, do the ironing, read a book, crochet (I'm addicted!). Do any activity that isn't looking at a mobile phone, TV or computer screen.
- Then, when you wish to go to bed, run a bath or shower. Drop a couple (literally—more will just overpower you!) of drops of lavender essential oil or an oil of your choice into the bath or base of the shower. Give your body time to relax. Breathe and practise "body gratitude."
- Notice how your sleep is: if you have worries that surface, jot them down in a journal or on a piece of paper (you can't do anything until the morning anyway), put them aside and allow yourself to unwind, prioritise sleep and then see how you feel. Learning new habits is not necessarily easy but once mastered it is well worth it.

CHAPTER 6

. . .

Worry and Boundaries

. . .

Can you recall the last time someone stepped all over your boundaries? Maybe you agreed to help out when you were, in fact, exhausted—and then felt more tired and also annoyed that you did not just say no? Saying no doesn't make you a bad person!

Maintaining healthy boundaries is paramount for a radiant woman. On an aeroplane, the flight attendant says that before helping anyone else with his or her oxygen mask, you should put your own on first. Every flight I have been on they say this. They do not say, "Put masks on everyone else around you and exhaust yourself, perhaps not even making it back to your seat." They do not say, "You are only worthy if you help others first so disregard your own needs entirely." No, they say, "Put on your own mask first." Perhaps there is a lesson for us?

I have a rule that I do not deal with work emails after supper. The modern world has allowed such boundaries to become blurred but I am adamant. All too often we let people intrude on us by telephone and email at all times of the day. Would you let someone waltz right in and sit down at your dinner table uninvited, disrupting your meal and your conversation? I hope not! Yet, that's exactly what we do when we bring mobile phones to the table and respond to calls or texts during dinnertime.

Learn to say no. That is easier said than done but it is perfectly okay to say "no". It is okay to answer the interruption or request with 'I am busy today. I can help you another day.' That is being true to yourself and also gives the other person the information they need to ask for assistance in the future.

Saying no is not being mean. It is not being lazy. Saying no is just clearly stating your boundaries. You have every right to do that. We all probably know people who are challenging to be around. Are you going to continue spending time with them, feeling anxious or unsettled, or do you recognise how you feel around them? If they are constantly negative, mean, unkind or manipulative (in your opinion or perception), then perhaps limiting the time you spend with them is wise.

I struggled with this a great deal; I would be with 'friends' even if spending time with certain people made me feel low or ill at ease. Tuning into how I felt allowed me to realise that I was utterly drained having seen certain people. I did not let this rule me but was grateful for this indication that something was not right. My husband pointed out to me that I don't have to be around people that drain me. I began to develop boundaries that allowed me to conserve my energy. I am now able to do so much more as I spend time with people that build me up, and I them, rather than feeling depleted and emotionally worn out. I find now I will actually leave the room or go for a walk if I am around those that are robbing me of my energy.

It is important to know what replenishes your energy levels (imagine you have batteries which are either filled up or drained by certain activities or by being around people) and adjust accordingly.

Perhaps you love silence but work in an environment that is very loud and noisy. Does that drain you? Are there alternatives to seek employment elsewhere? Or can you find ways to get time out, taking a lunch break outside for example. We can coast and ride the wave for a while but denying how you are feeling and how empty your battery is may catch up with you.

Perhaps the idea of maintaining or establishing a boundary is terrifying. I agree, I struggled with it for many years but there are some superb books on the subject and I will encourage you to head to the bibliography to learn more. Why not practise developing a boundary with little things first? Then you will gain the habit and experience in little things to know how to move on to larger issues and decisions.

Don't Worry...

... be happy! It took me a while to learn but once I embraced who I am today, it made life easier. Not perfect, just less pressure on me. I am enough for today and this stops me from worrying about tomorrow.

Today you are enough. Free up your thinking from worries and enjoy "enough" today. Simplistic as this sounds, it is liberating and gives rise to more freedom and clarity in your life.

I love this verse, "Has anyone by fussing in front of the mirror ever gotten taller by so much as an inch? All this time and money wasted on fashion—do you think it makes that much of a difference?" (*Matthew 6:27*)

I spent hours and hours fussing in front of a mirror, yet I did not believe in myself, which is a far more attractive feature than any expensive clothes or make up. Now, I am not saying don't brush your hair or put on nice clothes but letting these thoughts dominate your thinking is where the trouble lies. Worry can breed and take hold of your thinking.

You might say, "I can't do it." Fortunately God tells us we can learn to say, "I can do all things through Him who gives me strength" (*Philippians 4:13*). Nice to know, isn't it?

Some media would have us believe we are all doomed through daily reports of increasing health risks, natural disasters, epidemics of disease and wars. I do not wish to gloss over the fact. Many of these are going on right now and millions of people are suffering untold hardship in their lives. However, there is also a lot to be happy about. The trick is recognising that and focusing on the good and positive aspects of life rather than the negatives of doom and gloom.

Sadly, from my observations, negative news seems to fill the pages of newspapers, magazines and blogs more often than positive news does. Just think about our conversation topics too—positive or negative? It is surprising (once you become aware) of just how negative the news can be. Yet you can choose how much you wish to see and absorb. Whilst I think being entirely out of touch might not be wise, there is a limit to how much ghastly news you can handle.

I used to worry a lot; my Grandmother often said, "Joanna, why are you worrying? We are not."

My reply simply was, "Yes, Granny I am worrying, as no one else is."

Worry is like a rocking horse, though—it gives you something to do but gets you absolutely nowhere and can make you feel a little bit sick!

I was also someone who would say yes for a peaceful life rather than disagree or risk offending someone. Yet I simply hate it when someone appeases me or does something out of sufferance, so I was doing the very thing I find annoying! I would rather someone was actually honest than glossing over the truth. Honesty is the best policy!

We can work and worry too much. Perhaps you know that feeling? Constantly being connected, with your cell phone on at night and smart phone getting emails day and night, worrying about work when at the weekend there is not much you can do. The fight or flight response is there to protect us but, constantly activated, this can result in low-level stress and worry and this is certainly not good for our long-term health.[25]

One way to deal with the low-level stress you experience is what some call "sounding." Use sounding to go "aaaaaa" or "eeeee" or "iiiii"; that is a healthy response and may allow your body to remove some of the built up stress. I also find going on a walk where I can wave my arms, shake and hum makes a big difference to my stress level.

That is partly why I find a Nia class is so much fun; there is great music, sounding, you can laugh, cry, shout, giggle and wiggle—basically use your body in a more primal way by letting body awareness refresh your body, mind, spirit and emotions.

Modern stresses may be modern: deadlines, work commitments and the Internet not working. However, our body doesn't really know that; it is still programmed to deal with the threat of a lion or bear in the wilderness. A healthy response is to get angry rather than to suppress our feelings. It allows you to release the tension and pressure; the issue is what you do with that anger. Shouting at a tree rather than a family member is obviously healthy. Perhaps the old adage "take a deep breath and count to ten" can be useful too. I find putting on music and dancing helps enormously.

I think in society we (perhaps) incorrectly think anger is bad but actually it is very human. I am much more able now to recognise that someone who let me down made me feel angry and annoyed. I do not necessarily shout at them (obviously) but I am now able to verbalise how I am feeling, for example: "Ugh, I feel really annoyed; I feel so angry, let down and hurt."

I also cry a lot more than I used to. For years I would ignore my emotions and push them away rather than let on or admit (to myself) how I was feeling. The trouble is that pushing a spring (my emotions) down constantly took work and eventually I got burnt out and exhausted. It felt like having my foot on the accelerator and on the brake – do that in a car and you'll break it.

Now my feelings are much more short lived, i.e., I take things to the "rubbish bin in the sky" far more quickly than I used to. I keep short accounts. It is so liberating! I also refuse to go to bed angry. I will decide to put away whatever is bothering me and then see if I need to pick it up in the morning, or just let it go.

Worry is endemic in society today, "Aren't you worried about that?" I hear it regularly but as the years have gone by I worry less, mainly as my husband says to me:

"Joanna, can you do anything to change it?"

"No", I reply.

"Well, stop worrying."

He is right and I have learnt to hand it over, put it in the "rubbish bin in the sky" and use my powers for good!

Obviously there are still occasions where I do not have it all together and I think, "Ooh, what will I do", or, "How will I handle that?" Yet I know that nine times out of ten things work out and actually even if they don't go the way I thought, that is often a good thing!

GIVE IT A GO

- Next time you are tempted to get in a stew, stop. Tune in; notice how your body feels. What do your hands feel like, your jaw and your spine? Notice. Rather than getting all upset, ask yourself these questions: "Can I change it? Does my fussing and getting upset help me?" If the answers are "No", put each worry into the "rubbish bin in the sky".
- This may sound simplistic but many a poor decision has been made based on heat of the moment emotions, or a knee-jerk reaction to a worry or fear. "Well, why don't you sleep on it?" as my Mother says. That is another way to see what the healing nectar of rest, time and the subsequent clarity brings.
- John Steinbeck once wrote, "A problem difficult at night is resolved in the morning after the committee of sleep has worked on it." So why not give it a go?
- Write a list of the top stressors in your life. Divide into 'can do something' and 'let it go'—it might bring some clarity.

CHAPTER 7

. . .

Water, Fake Food and Real Food

. . .

You likely know that drinking water is a good idea? Yes? I hope so. There is much debate about how much to drink. Some make elaborate calculations but I think that means we end up drinking far too much, which can be just as damaging as not drinking enough. How much water do you drink? Eight glasses? I hope not, unless you are working in a hot desert somewhere!

My Mother is wise and always said have a glass of water before a pill. It often helped, not least, as I felt thirsty. For some, though, this mechanism has been overridden by relentless marketing and 'guidance' about drinking eight glasses of water a day. I got caught up in all the eight-glasses-of-water-a-day hype but all that did was give me a headache. I do not drink that much now. I have no headaches and have more energy, too.

Water is a marvelous, mysterious thing. Dr. Masuro Emoto's book *Hidden Messages in Water* shows quite astonishing photographs of water that formed different crystals after he exposed it to various words like "love", "beautiful", "peace" and "kindness". What he concluded was that water is affected by the words we say (as we are).[26] So, I will often bless the water I am drinking, saying something like, "Thank you, beautiful water, for nourishing my body." The water usually tastes pretty good! (And it's another good exercise in gratitude.)

Dr. Batmanghelidj's book, *Your Body's Many Cries for Water*, discusses how many of us consume fizzy drinks yet some of our recurrent health issues are due to dehydration. Dr. Batmanghelidj says that often, "you're not sick; you're thirsty. Don't treat thirst with medication."[27] Yet the dilemma is that many take things to *extremes*. Certainly there are some who could do with drinking more water but equally drinking too much water is highly unwise, too.

I drink a small glass of water when getting up in the morning; I will usually have a small cup of tea before breakfast. I love tea more so now that I am older. I have no idea why that is but tea is relaxing (for me at least) and it is rich in antioxidants. Yet, throughout the day, I simply drink when I am thirsty rather than a set amount as days vary. I tune in to what my body needs rather than forcing it.

If you drink lots of coffee you might get a headache if you try and give it up quickly. (Not ideal.) Drink a bit less if that is the case! Yet, some scientists have found that coffee protects you from all manner of ills.[28] Likewise, other scientists have discovered that tea has pretty fabulous features too.[29] Frankly, I think moderation is the key; if all you drink is tea and coffee then that might not be the answer, not least as caffeine reduces your ability to sleep.[30]

A radiant woman knows her own body and really the best way to see if drinking tea and coffee is serving you well is to ask your body. Do I feel good having tea and coffee in me all day? Or, if I am really honest, do I get a racing heart and feel better when I drink water instead? I am sure you know the answer; you just need to be honest and tune in long enough to listen to your body. Just because there are coffee shops on many street corners doesn't mean you have to have a coffee when you are passing!

Filter Your Water or Your Body Is the Filter

Bottled water is a huge business; billions of dollars[31] are made from this new industry that did not exist when I was a child. I find it bizarre to bottle water, ship it across the world and charge a premium price whilst creating tonnes of plastic bottles to clog landfill. It seems utterly crazy, or it is just me who has noticed? Yet bottled water is hugely popular. I see many people buying big bottles of water even though the water here in British Columbia tastes great and is safe. Reusable bottles and a home filter are a far more environmentally friendly way to go.

Needless to say, tap water is just fine; drink it and enjoy it—with a filter. Much of the tap water in North America and Britain is chlorinated and some fluoridated; there are arguments from both sides on these substances. Many say fluoride is great for our teeth; others say it is toxic waste. I don't waste my energy getting involved with the debate but I do filter my tap water. A filter is an investment and seeing as your body needs water, I think you are worth it. If water tastes palatable, I think it encourages you to drink it.

I would say that a water filter is a priority in terms of looking radiant; you are what you eat or drink so why not drink pure water? Bottled water, according to Annie Leonard in *The Story of Bottled Water,* is far less regulated than municipal water. Don't forget that in some cases bottled water can be ordinary tap water, so what you are buying is nothing more than filtered tap water in a plastic bottle. The tricky thing about plastic water bottles is that they can—if the plastic is #7[32]—potentially expose you to Bisphenol A, a synthetic chemical that is linked to hormonal disruption.[33]

There has been much media discussion about Bisphenol A; it is found in tin can linings and shiny thermal shop till receipts and is considered to be an "obesogen", a term coined by Bruce Blumberg.[34]

An obesogen is a synthetic chemical that has the ability to muddle with our hormones and upset the delicate balance of our body. Blumberg believes that many synthetic chemicals to which we are inadvertently exposed in our daily lives are, in part, contributing to the obesity epidemic.[35]

Good Wholesome Food

The obsession with advertising over new diets is rife in today's society. There are so many diet books out there, I am sure you have noticed. Eat this, not that, eat that not this, eat this on Monday but not on Tuesday. Eat like a bird and infuriate all your friends when you go round for supper.

I read an article in a Sunday paper that was jokingly discussing the writer's inability to organise a dinner party in Los Angeles. She is English (living in L.A. temporarily) and rather flippantly wrote on the email invitation, let me know what you do eat. The replies came thick and fast and were so varied that they were unachievable as there was little overlap. She decided to shelve the home dinner party idea and head to a restaurant instead! The restaurant could then have the fun of dealing with the no wheat, no gluten, no dairy, no meat, no sugar, no carbs, no fish, only low GI foods, no tomatoes or nightshades!

The trouble with all these popular diets is that something might work for one person but not for others. My suggestion, honestly, is eat like your great-grandmother or great-grandfather would have eaten. Eat like they did in the early 1900s: simple food and as close to nature as possible.

What this will do though (this comes with a warning!) is make you realise just how much modern food is processed. It is essentially commercially produced food for profit presented in jazzy packaging with debatable amounts of vital nutrients (sound familiar, like those glossy face cream boxes?). Food has changed, we now have claims on the packaging; I have never seen a cow with "low-fat" stamped on its backside, nor a chicken or carrot with "healthy" printed on it. I think a return to simple food is wise.

Butter or margarine? I eat butter and as Joan Gussow said, "As for butter versus margarine, I trust cows more than chemists."[36] I agree! Butter contains vitamins A[37], D, E[38] and K as well as the minerals iodine, magnesium, phosphorus and potassium.[39] Eating butter with vegetables can assist the absorption of the vitamins and minerals they contain—and makes it taste better too! Butter also has anti-cariogenic (tooth decay) effects.[40] That staggers me, as we have long shunned butter in favour of margarine; yet butter is natural, made from shaking cream and separating the buttermilk. You can even make your own butter (Recipe on page 92).

I can't help but wonder if butter got a bad reputation when actually the real issue with our food today is artificial syrups, artificial sweeteners and additives. I know I would far rather have meat, vegetables, or pasta and some butter than eat a modern "health" food that has modified this and synthesized that combined with some less than natural flavouring.

Would your Great Granny know what a powerful vegan snack bar was? If she is alive, why not ask her? I know my Great Granny did not use low-fat sauces or diet drinks. She ate real food: a roast joint of meat on Sunday with an apple crumble and fresh cream, then leftover potatoes and vegetable soup in the evening. The cold meat was served with a baked potato with vegetables for lunch the following day; any remaining meat was made into rissoles (mashed potatoes and very finely chopped meat and herbs) and fried for dinner with some fresh vegetables. Soups and bone stocks were staples. She did like a cup of tea (or two) in the afternoon with a little cane sugar and a ginger nut biscuit (or two). She was quite partial to baked beans but she did not drink or eat diet drinks and foods for the simple reason they were not available! She lived to 93 years old and died in her sleep of old age.

All the old people I know in their 80s and 90s eat real food. They think about their meals in advance; their version of fast food is a boiled egg and a slice of toast or a baked potato with cheese. They do not eat too much nor do they eat too little. They are still fit and trim; few are overweight.

Do you think they know something we're missing in our modern health-fad age?

Look Beyond the Label

Some foods available today are called "super foods"; they likely are super but so is real, simple food too. Quality vegetables, butter, pastured eggs, bone stocks, freshly-baked bread, soaked grains, herbs, fruit and pasture-raised meat can provide a superbly varied diet and be very nourishing. I am in favour of eating simply—why overcomplicate things? Let's not obsess over what we eat.

I love cooking and on moving to North America I found that diets were very different. Packaged foods were relied upon more whereas in the U.K. my friends all cooked from scratch. That is not always the case here.

I even make my own salad dressing; it takes three minutes and is really easy (Recipe on page 93). I would rather make my own at home than pay five dollars for a bottle of ready-made salad dressing that contains artificial additives, flavours and soya bean oil! A typical salad dressing's ingredients can be a variation of water, sugar, soy bean oil, white wine vinegar, salt, flavours and calcium disodium EDTA. (Keep reading to learn why soy bean oil might not be such a good thing.)

I think a lot of the new-fangled "label foods" are not something we need. There are some superb foods out there to which we did not have access forty years ago. However, I can't help but wonder if many of the new so-called health foods are simply slick marketing? "Organic", too, has become a buzzword that is bandied about but certifications and testing measures can only do so much. Some, perhaps wishing to take advantage of the popularity of anything organic,[41] cut corners; and conditions for animals or pesticide use vary hugely between the actual situation and consumer perception.[42]

I do buy foods in packets—it is challenge not to; organic pasta, oat cakes, lentils and baked beans (it's a British thing!) amongst others. You have to be alert as labels on packet foods may not necessarily reflect what is actually inside the packet! Words like pure, natural, good and delicious (according to whom?) can be used freely and for busy people, shopping in a hurry, this can lead to some unfortunate purchases.

Some foods, with lots of claims, could well be designed by marketing departments. How do I know? When I was at university I did a semester of food technology and packaging. We had to cook a food; in this case it was a tomato-based sauce for pasta. Then we had to perform every stage of production—from kitchen to shop shelf—within our class. The whole process involved rather less cooking than I thought (that was the easy part, actually). Most of the time was spent fiddling with infuriatingly small cardboard boxes and coming up with jazzy slogans for what really was, simply put, pasta sauce.

The tomato sauce ingredients were water, tinned tomatoes, modified starch, onion, garlic, mixed herbs, salt and pepper. What alarmed me was the adding of a teaspoon of modified starch and then lots of water. The small batch of tomato sauce became loads of tomato sauce. I had instantly increased my profits!

Perhaps labels on foods are nothing more than extraordinary marketing and advertising put there purely to get you to buy one product over another? As my Grandmother says, "Joanna, it is amazing what you can do with good advertising." How wise she is! Her views on diet drinks are hilarious. She says she might have the occasional can of normal fizzy cola pop after an exhausting day's fishing (she's in her 90s)! However, she adds, she would rather have sugar as she is never really sure what is in diet soda and the people she sees drinking diet drinks are quite often fat.

This view may not be as odd as you think. Helen Hazuda, a professor of clinical epidemiology at the Texas University School of Medicine, writes, "The promotion of diet sodas and artificial sweeteners may be ill-advised." Her studies found that the waists of those who drank two or more diet drinks a day grew six times as quickly as those who did not consume them.[43] Granted, the study did not look at other factors in a person's diet. Nonetheless it seems that diet drinks, despite being marketed as low in calories, may not actually help people to lose weight at all.

Aspartame is another ingredient in many foods and drinks today: colas, fizzy drinks, chewing gums, vitamins, cough syrups, snack bars, sugar-free drinks, sauces, salad dressings and many other processed foods. Aspartame has been widely discussed by Dr. Russell Blaylock in his book *Excitotoxins*. It is not easy reading but well worth the effort if you wish to know more about aspartame, monosodium glutamate (MSG), Parkinson's disease and Alzheimer's disease.[44]

Aspartame seems to affect the nervous system like MSG.[45] In the U.K. I avoid the additive known as E621, which is MSG and E951, which is aspartame.[46] So if you see on a packet these E-numbers, perhaps put them back on the shelf. In North America we do not have E-numbers. MSG can be hidden by words like autolysed yeast, flavouring and hydrolysed vegetable protein.[47]

I find MSG gives me a headache and the aftertaste of a diet drink or product with aspartame makes me feel quite unwell. Needless to say, in order to look radiant I avoid such artificial ingredients. No radiant woman wants a headache.

What Does It Take to Eat Better?

I love what Michael Pollan says in his book *In Defense of Food* (Penguin Books) about how we spend our time and money:

> **"While it is true that many people simply can't afford to pay more** for food, either in money or time or both, many more of us can. After all, just in the last decade or two we've somehow found the time in the day to spend several hours on the Internet and the money in the budget not only to pay for broadband service, but to cover a second phone bill and a new monthly bill for television, formerly free. For the majority of Americans, spending more for better food is less a matter of ability than priority."[48]

I could not agree more. We now all have mobile phones: mine is the lowest price it can be at $24 a month (I rarely use it at that), which is $300 a year. Add in our satellite television subscription, which is $58 a month or $696 annually, and that is nearly a thousand dollars on two things that are not vital to my existence. I therefore wonder if more of us actually could eat better but we would just rather spend our money and time elsewhere?

Perhaps it is due to the amount of time it takes to cook real food? We are sold images of 'simple, quick and easy' by saccharin-smiling people on the television when the truth of real food is that it takes time, chopping, boiling and washing up to create good food. I am in no doubt that it is worth it, though. My Grandmother still cooks food from scratch every day. She is happy, healthy and fit at over 90 years old! Others, who perhaps neglect the importance of sound nutrition, may not enjoy such robust health in their latter years. I would rather invest in my nutritional bank today to ensure continuing health tomorrow. If I neglect my nutrition today perhaps I will only regret it later?

The rise of new health foods is unbelievable. I can't help wondering if we had health foods all along but they just haven't been foods with trendy labels and large marketing budgets. As my Grandmother says, "We didn't have health foods; we just had food. Now I can't move in a supermarket for all the foods promising youth and longevity!"

My pick of the original, simple foods are:

- Fresh locally grown (or organic) vegetables (including potatoes) and fruits—a wide seasonal variety.
- Grass-fed meat (easy in Britain), local and or organic (get to know your local butcher or farmer and buy the best you can afford).
- Pastured eggs—not from cooped up, caged 'battery' hens but from those that can roam in the pen and eat bugs and see the sunshine. Keeping your own is fun but hard work.
- Fats and cold-pressed oils—butter, coconut oil, lard, beef dripping, cold pressed extra-virgin olive oil.
- Well-made bread and pasta with organic flour (if you prefer) and rice etc.
- Sweeteners like local honey, dark maple syrup and yes, even organic cane sugar - birthday cakes taste horrid without!
- Thoughtful cooking from scratch and three square meals a day.

The fact is that we need to eat, the list of foods above doesn't mean that is all you can eat, far from it! Food is such an emotive subject and everyone has an opinion on food. The easiest way to get into a very challenging argument is to have a party and invite your vegan friends along with those who make chicken liver pâté. Ask a leading question and watch the fireworks!

My own view on food (if you haven't picked up on it already) is to *keep it simple*. Life is complex and stressful enough without weighing beans or chicken breasts and creating enemies rather than friendships. I like Matt Stone's books for that very reason as he thinks many are obsessing over where their food comes from, whether it is "good" or "bad" when they would be better just eating food regularly and enjoying it.

A variety of food that we enjoy eating and which nourishes our body is what we need. Stress can affect our digestion[49] so stressing about what we are eating is unwise and important to avoid. Evelyn Tribole and Elyse Resch authors of *Intuitive Eating* say "Scream a loud 'NO' to thoughts in your head that declare you're 'good' for eating minimal calories or 'bad' because you ate a piece of chocolate cake."[50]

Perhaps you feel that real, local food is a luxury you can't afford? Let me assure you that eating well need not be expensive. Obviously, if you choose fillet steak everyday then yes, it will be very pricey. However, most people want chicken breasts not thighs, which means chicken thighs are cheaper. Fillet steak is pricey, as there is only a little bit in each animal, but stewing cuts are cheaper. Offal is barely used today but this oversight is a shame as there is valuable nutrition in chicken liver pate, for example. I love a stew with cheap cuts of beef or lamb. Add potatoes, vegetables and herbs and you have a nourishing hot pot.

Some restaurants use cheaper cuts of meat and make offal somewhat of a niche dish. If you are vegan then the very idea of this will likely horrify you but soy (or soya as it is called in Europe) horrifies me; let me explain why.

A great deal of our processed food stems from just a few common ingredients such as; corn, soya, canola (rapeseed in Europe), and beet sugar, yet I think a wider variety of daily foods is wise.

You would be absolutely amazed at how many processed foods contain soya; the label may not even say soya but rather something like hydrolysed plant protein or textured vegetable protein. Breakfast cereals often have soya in their ingredients. Then there is soya milk, salad dressings and sauces with soya oil. It is also in veggie burgers and many vegan foods are soya-based. The quantity of soya can add up to a lot in your diet. Even "healthy" snack bars often contain soya protein isolate. Soya is found in many fried foods, as soya oil is cheap for frying deep-fried foods.

But soya is a health food, isn't it? I'm not so sure. Soya can lead to heavy metal toxicity due to the packaging, as well as lowering minerals needed in our bodies for detoxification, according to Dr. Kaayla Daniel, author of *The Whole Soy Story*. Soya also has phytoestrogens, which are "plant oestrogens that are not identical to human oestrogens but are close enough to fool the body and cause significant endocrine disruption."[51] Remember, an endocrine disruptor essentially muddles your hormones.

A report by the Endocrine Society, discussing the role of endocrine disrupting chemicals, highlights that "natural chemicals found in human and animal food (e.g. phytoestrogens, including genistein [found in soya] and coumestrol) can also act as endocrine disruptors."[52] Furthermore, another recent study reported that "urinary concentrations of the phytoestrogen genistein... were about 500-fold higher in infants fed soy formula compared with those fed cow's milk formula."[53]

Perhaps you don't eat much soya. Or so you think. The tricky thing is that soy is often added to drinks, breads, sweets, snack bars and health food drinks. Recently in the UK I had to buy bread for my mother as we were making lots of sandwiches for a party. I looked at the ingredients of various loaves of bread; only two loaves out of the thirty on the shelves were made without soya flour! So just be mindful of how much soya you are actually eating or drinking.

I used to drink soya milk when I lived in the U.K. That was a very bad move—period pains like you would not believe and headaches.

Fortunately I was given a brochure called *Soy Alert* by someone my parents know, Jody Scheckter. That little brochure outlined research on the down side of soya. I realised it was not benefiting me and so gave up soya milk. I also learnt to scrutinise labels to avoid the insidious inclusion of soya in so many foods today.

One of the ways Kaayla Daniel suggests for healing the body after having eaten a lot of soya is making bone stocks. Making bone stock is a superb way to ensure you get nourishment without a hefty price tag (read on for directions how to make bone stock).

I have always thought we are wiser to eat nourishing wholesome foods rather than relying on vitamin pills to fill the gap of a junk diet. There is no end to the variety of vitamin pills you could take if you had lots of money and an hour in the morning to swallow them all!

Eat a Balanced Diet—There's Sense to This!

There is a reason that health professionals say, "Eat a balanced diet." Variety is the spice of life and it ensures we get a wide variety of nutrients. For example, fresh mushrooms grow in the fields and woods in autumn and they are rich in D vitamins,[54] which we need as the days get shorter and we are getting less sunlight. Pretty amazing isn't it?

Eating seasonally will very often ensure that you get foods with the vitamins and minerals that you need at a particular time of the year. When it is -4C (24F)—cold!—and I do not feel like eating salad, the idea of a warming soup or baked potato is far more appealing. In summer I feel like eating the bountiful lettuce, salad leaves and carrots that I grow in our garden. Nature is brilliant and, in most parts of the world, eating seasonal vegetables will ensure we get a good variety of nutrients throughout the year.

If you are fortunate to have a local butcher and greengrocer then ask for what you want. Supermarkets still have managers and they will order what customers want; it makes business sense! If you want a particular type of cheese or speciality item, just ask. Our local supermarket rarely had good quality beef bones for making bone stock. Then I asked for grass-fed, organic, beef bones, the manager got them in and now they sell lots of them. Just ask for what you want at your local shop.

Bone Broth Stock—What You Need to Know

I make bone broth stock most weeks; this is an old fashioned practice that is gaining popularity again. Making stock actually takes very little time to prepare. The hard work is done by your slow cooker or crock pot. I cook beef stock for two days and chicken for about twelve hours; this ensures a really rich stock and it is so easy to just leave in the slow cooker. Learn to make homemade chicken stock on page 94.

According to Dr. Natasha Campbell-McBride, creator of the GAPS Diet, "Meat and fish stocks provide building blocks for the rapidly growing cells of the gut lining and they have a soothing effect on any areas of inflammation in the gut. That is why they aid digestion and have been known for centuries as healing folk remedies for the digestive tract."[55]

I have found that my digestive issues have disappeared since I have incorporated bone stocks into our daily diet. I used to get such pain in my stomach from eating wheat, dairy and sugar products. Now I can eat pasta and digest it without any pain at all. I can also enjoy puddings and home-made jam again without a sore tummy! Bone stocks are amazing and there is a reason that many people around the world go to such lengths to make it.

My parents were in China on holiday a few years ago. Their guide and translator showed them the sites of the countryside around Shanghai and whilst they were there they went to a meat and vegetable market. The guide bought a live chicken, which was put in a bag in the boot (trunk) of the car. Whilst driving back to Shanghai my mother inquired why they had a live chicken in the boot, the reply came, "My grandfather is ill and very weak; chicken soup will revive and refresh him." The man intended to make chicken stock using the head, feet and neck.

This stock may seem unpleasant to some but having made stock using the feet of chickens, I can assure you the benefits are nothing short of miraculous! (Maybe there really is something to the home remedy for the common cold—chicken noodle soup—but I doubt it's the kind in a tin with soy protein isolate and mechanically separated chicken.)

Gelatine Jellies for Happy Nails and Skin

Jellies were a staple in our house when I was growing up. Mum used to make them in fun moulds; my favourite one was the tortoise mould! She did it because these easy-to-make, child-friendly puddings contain gelatine, which is rich in protein, some amino acids and collagen. These are all substances we need for strong hair, nails and skin as well as the joints and ligaments.[56] There are many expensive face creams containing collagen, but I prefer to eat my collagen since jellies are cheaper than collagen face creams!

Reap the benefits of jellies by making your own. I have included my recipe on page 96. Buying good quality gelatine is wise and I have listed places to buy it in the Appendix.

Be Grateful for Your Food

In their book *Abounding River*, Matthew and Terces Englehart conduct a great discussion about abundance—but the one thing that struck a chord in me was the encouragement to be grateful for food—and for those who grow, transport and prepare it. I personally believe that giving thanks for the vital labour of farmers and others is essential to being radiant. That thoughtful awareness sends more love into the world and we need that! Think back to a time when someone thanked you for something you did. It likely felt good, so why not give thanks to others?

I also personally believe that part of being grateful for our food means *eating* it! Skipping meals may feel appealing; the myth is that if you don't eat you'll lose weight. However, in many cases, skipping meals is not healthy. Breakfast is important, as you have not eaten since the evening before, hence you are breaking your fast. Depending on what time you ate supper the night before it can be over twelve hours that you have not eaten, yet many women today are inadvertently denying themselves daily. A grown woman cannot survive on limited calories for a prolonged period of time.

Some ideas for simple breakfasts are porridge (recipe on page 97), rice, bacon and eggs, toast and a boiled egg or yoghurt with fruit and some nuts. Eating something is wise. I find if I don't eat breakfast I get very hungry and do not think as clearly. Very often I will have the remains of supper for breakfast; who says you can't have spaghetti Bolognese for breakfast?

There are varying theories on how big our meals should be; some say we should breakfast like a king, lunch like a prince and dine like a pauper. However, you have to do what fits into your lifestyle. Needless to say, I feel better when I eat three proper sized meals a day.

I think we all know that food can be habit-forming, if not down-right addictive. So, if you are in the habit of snacking all day whilst not actually warranting the snack in terms of how much activity you have done, that is when it is useful to ask yourself, "How is this serving me?"

Don't be deceived; snacking attacks our waistline! In the last thirty years, snacking has become a regular pastime and many people eat far more than they need for daily activities.[57] No wonder clothing designers have had to increase the girth of women's clothes sizes.[58] Packets of potato crisps (chips) used to be about 35-40g, now they are huge grab bags[59]—and our bottoms and waistlines, in some cases, reflect this!

Snacking is a major profit earner for the food industry. *Snack Foods 2012*, a report by Keynotes says that the savoury snack industry in the U.K. grew by more than seven percent (7.1) in 2011, to reach an annual value of £2.71 billon.[60] A lot of marketing and advertising depends on getting us to eat more snacks. I can still remember the first television advert for a fudge bar in Britain in the 1980s. It had a catchy jingle and became the bane of my mother as I would see these bars when shopping and I would pester her. I am not sure I actually even liked them, as they tasted somewhat fake. I was old enough to know better but it shows the power of marketing catchy jingle tunes and the appeal of snacks. Snacks have come a very long way since then and are now available everywhere; newsagents, train stations, on trains, in aeroplanes, in hair dressers, you name it.

Whilst in London a few months ago, I bought a newspaper; the lady on the cash register said, 'Would you like to buy a chocolate bar for £1?' I said no thank you (the bar was huge, at least 250 grams of chocolate). I thought how strange that, in a country where obesity and overeating is a considerable burden[61] on the National Health Service, shops are enticing you to buy a large bar of chocolate when buying a newspaper.

Besides snacking, eating on the go is another totally accepted (negative) food trend these days. I would say that sitting down for meals as opposed to eating on the run is preferable. Call me old-fashioned but it allows you to consciously eat your food and perhaps gives more optimal conditions for the body to digest the nutrients in a more relaxed way.

Another aspect of proper regard for food lies in portion control. We don't want to be too greedy—or too stingy, or oblivious. I was in the habit of making food for my husband and myself and just halving the portions. Clearly that led to me putting on weight. I hadn't really thought about it. Now that I have got into the habit of my husband having two-thirds (he is a lot taller and bigger than I am) and my having one-third, I am back to a more normal weight for me—funny that!

When we were in the U.S.A. a few years go, my husband and I went to a nice restaurant and whilst looking at the menus glanced at the table next to us. The meal size was so big. We don't like wasting food so we ordered one meal and asked for two plates and were glad we did. The baked potato would have fed four of us; the salad was probably a whole lettuce and the steak was upsettingly large. We ate our supper. We had enough for a little lunch the next day, too. The bill arrived with a 20% discount. I queried this, not wishing to get the waitress into trouble if it had been incorrect. "Oh we gave you a discount as you couldn't afford to buy two meals" was her reply! I love their assumption but we simply didn't want to waste food. We gladly took the discount though! Portion size is an important variable to get right; not too much and not too little.

That said, at the other extreme there are those, as I said earlier, who are literally starving themselves and think they are just "eating healthily." A woman cannot survive on carrot sticks and hummus alone. Sometimes you just have to eat the croissant!

I have a family member who always has bitterly cold hands; she is an avid water drinker and is very slim. My mother on the other hand, is normal weight (and actually looks pretty incredible for being in her 60s!); she has warm hands, good skin and disposition—and she will not feel guilty having a biscuit at tea time. She eats a proper breakfast, lunch and supper. Some days she will open the cupboard mid-morning and have a few Brazil nuts, dates or a biscuit; she eats her three normal meals and, when necessary, a couple of little nibbles mid morning and mid afternoon only if hungry. I find that a good model.

Ayurvedic tradition suggests we eat in silence and have no distractions when eating. One study found that eating whilst distracted by for example television or talking on the phone resulted in those distracted subjects ingesting more energy / calories.[62]

Silence is fine if I am on my own but it's not overly sociable if my husband is around! I think seeking a happy medium is where the wisdom lies: eating whilst watching a violent television programme or being completely distracted, or stressed, is not great for digestion. Besides, pleasant conversation can be one of the best parts of meal times.

I recall when I was in Paris a couple of years ago, having lunch in a little bistro. We walked in at noon, sat down and gazed at the simple but delicious menu on the chalkboard. A lady was sitting next to us; she was drinking a small glass of water whilst reading the newspaper. Her food arrived: a piece of chicken, some dauphinoise potatoes and a salad. The waitress brought her a little glass of red wine, too. The lady put her paper away, paused and started to slowly eat her lunch. She was not reading or chatting—merely eating, chewing her food and watching the world go by.

In about 45 minutes she was finishing her lunch, which included a very small custard with fruit and an espresso coffee. She did not hurry, gulp, or stress whilst eating; she ate in silence and seemed to savour every mouthful. Then at 12.55pm she started to gather her (chic) coat, her newspaper and her umbrella. She stood up, brushed down her clothing and walked out of the bistro. Her lunch hour was peaceful. She savoured her food. Her face, whilst not young, was truly radiant. She paused within her day long enough to "smell the roses" or, in this case, her delicious Parisian bistro lunch!

How is your lunch hour? Is it rushed, hurried and stressful, or is it more serene and peaceful? Do you eat at your desk all stressed or perhaps in front of the television or playing with your tablet or telephone? Do you feel this is conducive to optimal digestion? I ask this question of you certainly not to lay judgment (far from it as I spent years eating like this and had terrible tummy aches). I merely raise this so you are aware of it. It may (or may not) be something you wish to change.

We all need to eat to survive. The difference is that many of us eat far, far too much food that contains huge amounts of sugar and, more recently, high fructose corn syrup (HFCS). HFCS, is also called glucose-fructose syrup in Europe.[63] There is much negative press about HFCS; so much so that there have been moves in North America to re-brand HFCS as "corn sugar" (perhaps in the hope that that sounds more appealing) but the Food and Drug Administration vetoed that in 2012.[64]

I have cut back on consumption of sugar and sweet foods. Obviously, eating a normal western diet means that avoiding sugar completely is practically impossible. That said, reading labels is essential and sensible.

Sweetness is added to so many foods, even so-called healthy foods. By reading labels you'll see the true extent of where the sweet treats hide:

- Sugar
- Glucose-fructose syrup
- High fructose corn syrup
- Evaporated cane juice

The concern I have is it seems every item you eat these days has sweetness in it: breakfast cereals, coffee milk substitute (I tried it once but didn't see the point!), bread, salsa, sandwich fillings, meats, smoothies, sauces, pasta bakes, ready made meals, fast food and obviously desserts and puddings. Wild over-consumption of sugar is when issues can arise. The average American eats nearly 152 pounds of sugar a year;[65] that is more than my whole body weight in sugar! The average Canadian eats 26 teaspoons of sugar a day.[66] The average person in Great Britain eats 238 teaspoons a week.[67]

Average sugar consumption in teaspoons per day:

Canada:	26
United Kingdom	34
United States	40

(Calculations based on figures quoted above).

Curb Sugar Cravings with Fermented Foods

One way to curb sugar cravings is to eat fermented foods, according to Donna Gates co-author of *The Body Ecology Diet*. I attribute part of my success in kicking the sugar habit to eating a small amount of fermented foods with meals. These fermented foods include sauerkraut, kimchi, kombucha and good quality milk yoghurts amongst others things. Eating these foods, as part of a varied and balanced diet is one way to maintain a happy digestion and efficient bowels.[68] Bear in mind that this doesn't mean eat oodles of yoghurt or kimchi. Moderation! One of the silliest things we can do is when we hear "X" is good for us is we only eat "X". Balanced diet is the sensible choice.

Donna Gates says, "Once you add fermented foods and drinks to your diet, you will soon lose your desire and cravings for sweet foods."[69] I actually emailed Donna to ask her more about fermented foods and sugar, this is what she said:

"Within each of us is miraculous inner ecosystem which is the key to vibrant health. Cultured vegetables are essential to restore its balance, control sugar and carbohydrate cravings, improve overall digestion and elimination, cleanse toxins, strengthen your immune system and rejuvenate your cells. Fermented foods will guide you to a younger, healthier, happier you."[70]

I found exactly that. I thoroughly enjoy a croissant, cake or jam on toast but I don't crave them; in fact I am relatively ambivalent towards them. By contrast in my twenties I would crave sweets, pasta, cakes and any sweet food I could find. Years later, craving sugar seems so alien to me. Our metabolism can change!

The humble cabbage holds an impressive secret when fermented. Most would say cabbage is dull when boiled but if you crush it raw and add sea salt and time you get amazing sauerkraut. Sauerkraut is a great addition to any modern diet and it is surprisingly easy to make (recipe on page 98). It is rich in live bacteria and probiotics[71] which we need for digestion and for our immune system. According to Gary B. Huffnagle of the University of Michigan, "...probiotics do much more than promote the health of our gut. They also foster profoundly important changes in our white blood cells. That means an immune system that serves us, rather than harms us."[72]

As a side note, I want to comment on the relentless marketing campaign that has led us to believe in the preference for an antibacterial existence. A completely sanitary existence appears to be doing us more harm than good. Mark McMorris, M.D., a pediatric allergist at the University of Michigan Health System, says, "We've developed a cleanlier lifestyle and our bodies no longer need to fight germs as much as they did in the past. As a result, the immune system has shifted away from fighting infection to developing more allergic tendencies."[73] Is the trending rise in allergies due to over-zealous cleaning and spritzing with antibacterial sprays? Quite possibly.

Bacteria are the essence of life; a child at birth (assuming it's a natural delivery) gets some of its gut flora from its mother, then breast milk and later enzyme-rich, real food provides more beneficial bacteria. If a diet of processed foods is favoured, the necessary bacteria are lacking.

Today, sauerkraut and other fermented foods are enjoyed in many countries throughout the world, in particular Russia, Germany and

Poland. Kimchi, fermented cabbage with chili and fish sauce, is eaten in Korea. I adore kimchi and feel that dismissing fermented foods from our diet is unwise. I made a superb batch of kimchi recently using the recipe from Alex Lewin's book, *Real Food Fermentation*, which is a great reference for all things fermented (I adore the preserved lemons and limes recipe).[74]

Healthy Thoughts about Sugar

Traditionally we would have eaten fruit in summer when it ripened on the tree or bush, we might have a glut of apples, raspberries or black-berries. Now with modern food preservation and transportation we are able to get fruit all year round. Deep freezes mean we can have raspberry sauce in December, should we wish. I recently met a fruitar-ian, someone who *only* eats fruit! There are extremes indeed and I do not think it is healthy or sensible.

**The secret to a radiant diet is finding
relaxed balance around food.**

As you know, too much of anything is unwise because it is unbalanced. The low-fat fad is rife and many low-fat foods actually contain lots of sugar or even artificial additives and sweeteners. Low-calorie might be low-calorie but perhaps we are looking in the wrong place? Surely we are wise to look at ingredients rather than attractive claims of 'good for us', 'low calorie' or 'with added fibre'.

Awareness is the key!

My dentist says if you are going to eat sweets do it in one go and then clean your teeth. I can still recall being allowed two sweets after lunch as a child. It was such a treat! Very often, I would save them to eat later which in theory was fine but my plan was not well thought out; unfortunately my hiding place was also somewhere that the resident mouse family went, so more often than not my sweets were eaten for me! That is one of the joys of growing up in a very old house in England; there are many nooks and crannies in which to (not always successfully) hide things.

Another writer on the topic of sugar is John Yudkin. In his book *Pure, White and Deadly* (out of print for years until a reissue print in December 2012) he discusses the topic of chronic diseases (like cancer and heart disease), which he felt might be exacerbated by sugar and not (as many still believe) the much-demonised saturated fat. Yudkin argues that sugar is, in fact, the main problem with our modern diets rather than saturated fat.[75] This stands to reason; we quite likely eat less saturated fat than we used to with such relentless butter bashing in doctors' offices and the media. Think about how many of us used to eat butter and now we deny ourselves, opting instead for a plastic tub filled with vegetable oils and flavourings.

Whilst denying ourselves saturated fat and 'naughty' butter, we choose to eat foods containing oodles of sugar. Yet, the nation is not getting any thinner (and one could argue healthier). Have we incorrectly demonised butter and lard when actually sweetness and indulgence is the issue?

Sugar was once a luxury and my mother remembers when she was a child in England and sugar was rationed. So, for weddings and birthday cakes, friends had to club together to pool their sugar rations. I can't help but wonder that today's over indulgence is just from sugary sweet foods being so readily available and relentlessly marketed at us 24 hours a day.

Sugar is also thought to disrupt the skin in a process called *glycation*.[76] I have youthful skin and often people do not believe I am really 38 years old. However, I do not rely on sugary foods as staples in my diet.

I do occasionally enjoy a croissant, bread and jam, or a homemade slice of cake but the key word in that is *occasionally*; not all day every day.

But be under no illusions, I *enjoy* the sweet treat when I eat it. Where is the joy in guilty eating? If you are going to have a slice of cake, then eat it and enjoy it! Life is, after all, for living; just use moderation.

There will always be strong opinions on diet and that is precisely why I have not given you tonnes of recipes and strict recommendations. Just as you can buy processed, sweet-tasting foods doesn't mean they are wise to buy day in and day out.

Find out what works for you. Don't do yourself a disservice and say you don't know. You do; tune in and listen!

Why not start to eat a little fermented food every so often, just a teaspoon here and there, not necessarily every day but just see how you feel? You might fart a bit initially; forgive me for being basic but at least you know!

Ask yourself, what are you really eating? Are you nibbling at things here and there, like a grazer, and never sitting down to a proper meal? How do you think you'd feel if you ate three good meals a day? You could try it and see! The tendency to snack may lessen.

Eating nutrient-dense food such as the simple foods I have discussed along with adequate amounts of beneficial fats like coconut oil for example may well ensure you are not so hungry between meals. I eat more fat now than most doctors might be happy with. The common medical view is that fat is bad and some undoubtedly are. I do not eat trans-fats and many vegetable oils. However, I believe we do need fat in our diet.

You need food (fuel) for energy! Think of a fire. It can burn well but if you do not put another log on the fire it goes out. Many women desire to be slim but they're not putting enough logs on their fires, so to speak—and so are not eating enough, which Matt Stone, author of *Eat for Heat,* believes has a detrimental effect on our metabolism. It is a delicate balance.

Get to Know Your Bowels

Bowel activity, whilst not the most polite subject to discuss at a dinner party, is a topic that is actually very important to our radiance and over all well being.

It has been said, "It is not what a woman eats so much as what she can digest that matters… The blood cannot be pure if the body is not fed properly, washed regularly and given sufficient exercise."[77] I would add that by exercising and eating well you are removing toxins and waste.

Going to the bathroom is something we all need to do. Putting food in has to result in taking something out at some point. Detoxing is important. (You know that by now but I am not talking pricey green detox drinks here; I am talking easy-to-do daily detoxing by simply visiting the bathroom.) One of the easiest ways to detox is through daily bowel movements.

It isn't necessarily very ladylike to be chatting about bottoms and poo but it is vital to understand that if you eat and don't poo then that isn't very balanced. Toxins can build up in your body and make you feel less than optimal and lead to dull skin and aches and pains. One study found that infrequent bowel movements were associated with an elevated future risk of Parkinson's disease[78]; could this mean that we are not naturally (and easily) detoxing each day?

Perhaps you have even bought expensive detox drinks, kits and herbs? Yet, if you are eating *occasional* fermented foods, taking exercise and eating regular meals and having regular bowel movements, then you will very likely be detoxing daily. Every time you visit the bathroom you are (to a greater or lesser extent) detoxing.

The benefit of healthy bowels is that you are detoxing gradually rather than once a year enduring a hellish week of eating nothing but lettuce! Obviously I am joking, but I am not a fan of these types of regimes; where is the joy in that? Some swear by them and happy days if they enjoy it. I'd rather just eat well, laugh, go for a walk, drink some water and use the bathroom regularly than endure weeks of greenery in a glass whilst feeling hungry and cold! It is all about tuning in and eating intuitively if you like; some days I feel like a salad for lunch, other days I feel like a hearty soup, perhaps I feel like an egg sandwich. Variety seems to serve me well.

GIVE IT A GO

- Start to read labels on food. The first ingredient is the largest proportion of the food. Are you paying for water or sugar as the first ingredients? Labels are your friends; they show you what is in your food, usually!
- Enjoy your food, realise that you need to eat to live. Feeling guilty about whether your food is good or bad is unproductive. Slow down whilst eating; make meal times a special time when you are not multitasking. Simply eat and enjoy it, guilt-free. A biscuit is not bad in itself, though living on them is unwise!
- Consider adding a fermented food into your diet and see how you get on. Start slowly. One teaspoon might be good; that doesn't mean eating a whole tub is better! You can buy unpasteurised sauerkraut, if you are nervous about making it yourself.
- Always opt for the best-quality food you can afford. Food is your fuel and is worth investing in.

Butter

INGREDIENTS:
A pot of double cream (heavy cream), at room temperature.
A litre mason jar or a big jam jar.

METHOD:
Pour the cream into the jar; put the lid on FIRMLY!

Shake the cream in the jar for ten minutes.

You'll notice that the cream goes through stages; it first looks like it has curdled then there will be a lump of the forming butter. As you keep shaking you'll see more buttermilk (milky water-like) substance.

Put ice cubes in a bowl. Squeeze the butter ball under a cold running tap. (You are aiming to squeeze out as much butter milk as possible). Keep squeezing the butter under the cold tap. Roll the butter into little balls and place in the iced water.

Either keep the little butter balls in a jar or put all the butter in a butter dish. This will last about a week in the fridge. Making butter is really that simple!

How to Make...

Salad Dressing

INGREDIENTS:

50mls apple cider vinegar

150mls extra-virgin olive oil

1 tsp Dijon mustard

1 tsp dried mixed herbs

A little squirt of tomato puree

Good pinch of salt and a few grinds of pepper

METHOD:

Mix in a jam jar or pretty bottle with a tight fitting lid.

Shake well.

Easy peasy!

Homemade Chicken Stock

INGREDIENTS:

Chicken carcass   Parsley
1 onion   Celtic sea salt
2 cloves of garlic   Freshly-ground black pepper
2 carrots   Apple cider vinegar
Celery stick

METHOD:

Buy a good quality pastured or organic chicken (if you can)—don't worry simply buy the best quality you can afford. After roasting the chicken and removing the meat to eat for meals, save the carcass and pull off all the bones, including any remaining little bits of meat. Put it all into a slow cooker or crock pot. Roughly chop and add the vegetables. Finally add a generous sprinkle of Celtic sea salt and freshly ground black pepper.

Then (this is the important part!) pour in a tablespoon or two (max) of apple cider vinegar—this helps to draw the minerals from the bones and makes bone broth an easy way to get minerals and also gelatine.[79] It is ideal if you have a family member who is unwell or has a delicate constitution.

Leave everything cold in the slow cooker for an hour before heating. Turn the setting to high initially with the lid on. There may be scum that rises to the top; if you wish you can skim this off. Once the stock is bubbling you can leave it on low for the day (if you started in the morning) or overnight (if you make it in the evening). Once you have cooked it for at least seven hours, leave it to cool.

Get a large bowl or glass canning jars that will fit in the fridge. Use a sieve and funnel to strain the bits out of the stock and pour the stock into the jars or bowl. Store in the fridge if you are going to use it in the next couple of days. If not, pour it into ice cube trays and freeze it for later use in soups, sauces and stews. A layer of fat will form on the top of the stock, which you can discard or use for cooking.

You can also make stock in an oven proof saucepan; Le Creuset® is ideal. You can make it the same way as the slow cooker method but just bring to the boil on the hob and then put in a low oven (to simmer) for four or five hours.[80]

One of my favourite ways to use stock (other than chicken and sweet corn soup) is to make an easy mug of soup for lunch: add a few frozen stock cubes to a little pan, add some water, bring to the boil and boil for five minutes, then add a slice or two of spring onion, or garlic, salt and pepper and mixed herbs. Drink it like a shop-bought powdered soup—without the colours, additives or MSG!

How to Make...

Jellies

This makes six little jellies or three big jellies.

INGREDIENTS:
2 tsp good quality gelatine
3-4 tsp sugar
325mls hot water
140g fruit
Small glass jars or ramekins
Measuring jug and spoons

METHOD:
Boil the kettle. Put a little fruit in the bottom of the glass jars. Pour the hot water into the measuring jug. Sprinkle the gelatine on top. Set aside for five minutes to allow the gelatine to melt.

Once melted add the sugar. Stir to ensure the gelatine and sugar are fully mixed into the water.

Gently pour on top of the fruit in the glass jars.

Put in the fridge to cool.

HOW TO MAKE...

Porridge

INGREDIENTS:

½ cup of rolled oats, steel cut, not instant, per person (adult) per serving

2 ½ cups of filtered water, per person

1 teaspoon fresh lemon juice

METHOD:

Soak oats over night with lemon juice and water.

Warm slowly, stirring regularly on a low heat, until oats are tender.

Serve with fresh cream, honey or maple syrup, some fruit and nuts such as hazelnuts or sunflower seeds. I also like to add a little coconut milk or shredded coconut, if I have some available.

How to Make...

Fermented Cabbage (Sauerkraut)

Ingredients:

2 one-litre glass-canning jars
1 medium cabbage - remove green outer leaves and core
1tbsp – 1.5tbsp Celtic sea salt
Cocktail muddler - if available
Glass bowl
A little filtered water

Method:

Make sure the equipment and your hands are clean as per normal cooking procedures. Please avoid antibacterial dish soap as you need bacteria to ferment the cabbage!

Shred or chop cabbage, put in the bowl, sprinkle with salt; this starts the fermentation!

Now the fun, messy part: Pound cabbage with the muddler or crush and squeeze with your hands but not if you are wearing nail polish which can chip into food. Squeeze liquid from the cabbage. This takes about ten minutes.

Put sauerkraut into jars. Push firmly into the jar; you are removing air bubbles. The liquid will be level with the top of the cabbage. If it is not, add some filtered water. Keep on the kitchen bench, temperature between 15-25 C (59-77 F).

Roll the jars daily. Carefully, open and close the lids daily; they will go "pssst!"

After about six to eight days, put jars in the fridge.

Enjoy eating it with meals but if you have never had sauerkraut before start with a little bit; a teaspoon is enough. Too much might mean you fart rather a lot!

If you wish to jazz up the sauerkraut then why not make kimchi? The only difference is that you will add some chili flakes, garlic, ginger and a little fish sauce. Watch out, though, as some fish sauces contain monosodium glutamate (MSG or E621)—so read the labels carefully.

PART TWO

...

External Care

of the

Radiant Woman

...

CHAPTER 8

. . .

Exercise, Sunshine and Care of the Eyes

. . .

In the United Kingdom, the average person walks or cycles for just 11 minutes a day![81] A recent report in *The Lancet* said inactivity is now causing as many deaths as smoking. Report co-author Dr. I-Min Lee said, "Being inactive increases your risk of developing chronic diseases."[82]

It is easy to become a victim of inactivity. In Canada the average amount of time spent on the Internet, according to web research firm ComScore, is 43.5 hours a month![83] That is a lot of sitting still, simply using a mouse at the computer or your eyes whilst reading. Inactivity is a growing issue and it is not just Dr. I-Min Lee that thinks it can have an impact on diabetes and heart problems. Dr. Marc Hamilton, Ph.D., professor of biomedical sciences at the University of Missouri says "If you can perform a behaviour while sitting or standing, I would choose standing."[84] I know women who have treadmill desks; I'm not there yet!

It's not as difficult as you might think to get good exercise every day. Many of my girlfriends in London are savvy and have not joined a gym but they walk to work. By doing this they are walking a couple of miles twice a day. They walk in their trainers and put on their smart shoes once they are at the office. This incidental exercise is part of their day, saves them money on tube fares and gym memberships and keeps them trim.

Regardless of how you get it, daily exercise is vital. Exercise is how the body stimulates the lymphatic system and it also encourages bowel movements and brightens the skin. (A sluggish body can give rise to dull-looking skin, among other things.) Exercise can include gardening, bicycling to the store, walking up the stairs instead of taking the lift or going for a brisk walk around the block in your lunch hour. I highly encourage you to get outside or walk each day.

Exercise can lift your mood and improve your skin. You will feel warmer after a walk as you have stimulated the circulation. It is easy to feel cold sitting at a desk or not moving much but through exercise you get the blood pumping around your body and you will very likely feel warmer. I feel dreadful if I don't go for a walk each day. I don't run (unless I am late for the bus) but I do walk briskly with determination. I have a fabulous bubble umbrella that keeps me dry in the rain and I have a variety of gumboots, shoes and snow boots to suit all the weather we get here in western British Columbia. Even though I often do not remotely feel like going out for a walk, I still do and am glad of it.

Spend Time Outdoors

One of the benefits of being outside is that it allows you to hear the birds, see the sky and feel the sun and fresh air on your skin. Being in nature calms the mind and in our exceptionally busy world that is a very good thing. The sunshine on your face, in particular your eyes, helps to set your internal clock.[85]

The last twenty years have seen many people become very fearful of the sun, which I feel is a shame as having a sensible relationship with the sun is one of the great joys in life. Is it fear-based marketing, a desire to sell more lotions and potions, or is the sun really as dangerous as many say? I used to use oodles of sun cream. I am sure we can all remember being slathered in cream by a well-meaning adult? It was not until a decade ago that I even stopped to think what was in the thick sun cream that smelt so strong! Curiously, whilst wearing sun cream I still burnt. I was staying in the sunshine for hours and hours hoping that the cream would protect my pale English complexion. It did not!

Have you ever stopped to read the ingredients of the tubes of cream we (and our children) slather liberally on our skin? I have to wonder what is worse—the rays of the sun or the ingredients in sunblock! I avoid oxybenzone and retinyl palmitate.[86] A growing number of manufacturers use nano-particles (zinc oxide and titanium dioxide for example) and this is a cause of much controversy. A 2004 Royal Society report on nanoparticles stated, "We recommend that the ingredients lists of consumer products should identify the fact that manufactured nanoparticulate material has been added."[87] I haven't seen such labeling—have you?

Sunscreen is only a relatively recent invention but we spend millions and millions of dollars, and pounds, each year on it. The sun is an emotive subject of much debate; does it cause harm or not? Using common sense in the sun is my solution. I would rather wear a shirt and enjoy the shade of a peaceful tree than slather on strong-smelling lotion with lots of ingredients. If you burn then seek shade. I can't go on a tropical holiday armed only with bikinis, I have to seek shade — common sense really!

The sun actually helps us make Vitamin D and, according to *The New Home Encyclopedia* (written in 1932), exposure to sunlight is best done in a hot, shady spot. So it seems "sun-bathing" in the past was not done in direct sun. Is it any wonder we burn by lying on a sun bed by the pool?

Vitamin D levels have fallen in Europe in recent years; is this due to our use of sun cream? Along the same line, rickets cases are now more common in Great Britain.[88] Could that be due to our desire to avoid the sunshine? Is it due to children having computers and not wanting to play outside? Again, sensibility is the key.

Some sun-wise tips:

- **Get outside and enjoy some sunshine!** Don't be afraid of enjoying the sun just be sensible; obviously don't lie on a sun bed or lounger at 12 noon with only baby oil on—that's oh so 70s!
- **Go out in the sun before noon or after 3pm** if you are gardening or taking a long walk (i.e., any activity where you are out for longer than 30 or so minutes). Be mindful of how long you spend in the sun, if you have very pale skin.
- **Before I go into the sun I put *shea butter* on my skin.** This is not a sun cream as such but I find it helps my skin when in the sun. Shea butter is rich in vitamin E. If you buy shea butter please buy fair trade (see Appendix for ideas).
- **Clothes are a safe way to enjoy being outside on sunny days;** so are hats and shady trees! Look at animals—they rarely lie out in the blazing sun at midday, they usually seek shade, or a combination there of.
- **If you have to be in the sunshine all day and it is blisteringly hot, consider finding an eco-friendly sunscreen.** I like the Miessence Outdoor Balm (for more details see Appendix).

In very hot weather, curiously I find a cup of tea very refreshing. Tea contains some *antioxidants,* as do fresh fruits (including tomatoes) and vegetables, which play a role in healthy skin. Professor Mark Birch-Machin, of the Department of Molecular Dermatology at Newcastle University in Great Britain, says, "We know an antioxidant-rich diet is important as part of overall sun protection, but eating tomatoes will not make you invincible".[89]

Doctors in the UK have actually recommended gardening and outside time for those who are feeling low or depressed before relying on pharmaceutical drugs. According to Sir Richard Thompson, president of the Royal College of Physicians, time spent planting and pruning can be more powerful than a dose of pricey pills. He says, "Drug therapy can be really expensive, but gardening costs little and anyone can do it."[90] Sir Richard is a patron of Thrive, a national charity in Great Britain that provides gardening therapy.

When out for a walk, stop for a moment and just breathe in the world. Notice the sights, sounds and smells. Many people complain about the rain or the snow but the weather is one thing that we have no control over, so why not just enjoy what the day gives you? By walking every day you will likely notice that you can walk further with more ease. If you are unfit today, don't worry, take a small walk and then increase the length; Olympic athletes are not born gold medal winners. Start your walking regime with one step and another; ten minutes a day, then fifteen, then half an hour; it really is that simple. Remember, we all start somewhere, why not start now?

However You Do It, Get Moving!

I found when writing this book, if I got "writer's block", I would do the Nia 5 stages and the clarity returned. How can this be so effective? We were never designed to be static, sitting at a desk for hours on end. Our bodies like to move and if we do not move that is when we stagnate, get tired, become irritable and feel blurry. Just look at a child or a dog;

they sleep, granted, but they also move and change positions, use their body and stretch by exploring through life. We as adults need to do this—not as something nice to do but need to do.

Think how many times you ache, are feeling stiff, or wish you had more flexibility. Many issues in old age can be alleviated often through regular exercise. I say this as I know first hand; whilst writing this book I would sit at my desk for hours. I would lose myself in writing, editing and moving things about the page. The result? Stiffness. I truly felt old. Some mornings I would wake up cramped and stiff. Fortunately, I knew straight away why and so I made myself do the Nis 5 Stages first thing in the morning, use the MELT method (more on that later) or some days take a walk in the morning. I found I could get far more done in a shorter time having had fresh air and some movement. I often do more Nia 5 Stages in the evening. The result? Good sleep and no more achy feelings.

Shake It!

You have likely seen a dog having a good shake and wiggle? Dogs love a good stretch after they have been sleeping or lying in one position. We are no different and sitting still at a desk for hours a day is not conducive to feeling fabulous all day, unless you take a few minutes throughout your day to shake, wiggle and stretch.

Don't laugh! It may look (and feel) odd but there is a great deal of value in physical "jerks" like skipping or hopping around the room, or standing on one leg and then the other. These simple exercises are very easy to do. They are free, simple and a good way to maintain balance and coordination.[91]

To use wiggling as a way to get the body moving throughout the day, stand up and sense your feet. Then relax your jaw and start to gently shake and wiggle (imagine that you are shaking like when you are cold/freezing, or dancing to some frenetic music). Shake for about 30 seconds; perhaps imagine that someone is tickling you! You might find that you feel more energetic. I find this stimulates the body and brings more mental clarity.

Seven-Minute Daily Workout

This is based on the Nia 5 Stages but is very quick and remarkably fun to incorporate into your life. You spend one minute in each of the Nia 5 stages, all done on the floor.

Embryonic: Fluid-like, circular, rolling about on your back, front and sides. Relax your jaw and, when ready, move to the second stage.

Creeping: Lizard-like, one hand long in front of you and the other near your shoulder; one leg long and the other leg bent, creeping along the floor. When ready, move to crawling.

Crawling: Cat-like, on all fours, head looking out at the world in front of you. Relax your jaw; eyes are open to see your future. When ready, move to standing.

Standing: One foot flat on the floor, the other foot on the toes, relaxed. Arms are by your side or reaching out. Your eyes are able to look all around you. Move from one foot flat on the floor to the other. When ready, stand up and move into the final stage.

Walking: Tall spine, feet flat on the floor, eyes open with your jaw relaxed. You are standing, hands by your side. Notice the length of your spine, the stability in your feet. Take a few steps around the room; each step you are further from your past, walking into your future.

Next in the Seven-Minute Workout, get up and down from the floor; this can be done slowly or quickly. Do this for one minute. Up and down. Stand up and then get down onto the floor. If you need to modify this activity; sit in a chair and rise to standing in different ways.

The final stage is laughing: on your belly, then on your back, whilst squatting and then standing. Laugh out loud. (In Chapter Nine you'll find out why laughter is included in the Seven-Minute Workout.)

Breathe and Move

Remembering to breathe is also important, obviously! You may chuckle and think I'm being overly simplistic but many of us breathe very shallowly[92] and our body and brain need oxygen. Some deep, peaceful breaths outside first thing in the morning can refresh you and really start your day well. If you have been sitting at a desk for a few hours venture outside and take a few deep breaths, it will likely refresh your body and brain.

It does little good to be inactive. Think of a pond versus a river: one is static and one is roaring movement and has the ability to carve gorges. You have no doubt heard the phrase, "Use it or lose it"; well, it is true. I know athletes nearby that have had horrific injuries. They've had broken bones and all manner of injuries that prevented them from exercising the way they did prior to being injured. Do you think that stopped them in the long-term? Not at all! They were counting down the days until they could get back to walking, cycling, skiing or hockey and moving their body.

Here's something to try: Next time you are in a really bad mood, get down on the floor and move. Roll on your back. Sense your toes, the cheeks of your face. Are you gripping your jaw? Tap into your body sensations and be in the present. Let your body move and focus on relaxing rather than gripping your jaw being angry. I find when I am in a bad mood it helps to bring perspective!

You could also go for a gentle walk, breathing in the fresh air and looking away far into the distance, then close up and into the distance again; get the eyes moving! Your eyes will thank you for it too; they dislike static planes of vision, so staring at a computer screen for hours on end is not conducive for great vision.[93] If you can, look away from your computer screen at least every twenty minutes; it may just be out the window, or to the far end of the office. Focus on a dot on the wall and then come back to looking at your desk. Eyes are like everything else in our body; use them, treat them well and they, very likely, will be happy. Again, it is a matter of "use it or lose it".

Care of the Eyes

According to Dr. William H. Bates, "The fact is that when the mind is at rest nothing can tire the eyes and when the mind is under strain nothing can rest them. Anything that rests the mind will benefit the eyes."[94] Our eyes are worth protecting.

The New Home Encyclopedia claims that, "Blinking and winking are good movements for the eyelids, although the habit is one to guard against at unsuitable times". (No inappropriate winking at strangers no matter how good it is for your eye muscles!)

Perhaps consider finding a Bates Method practitioner.[95] I work with a lady who tests my eyes every month and the funny thing is that she can tell when I am stressed as my eyes are not as sharp. So, if you are stressed, perhaps going to the optician for your annual check-up at that time isn't wise; it might cost you a bit more in designer glasses!

Palming is a good way to relax the eyes and facial muscles[96] and I have noticed an improvement in my overall vision and awareness whilst easing eyestrain. Our days can be very long and visually demanding; "eyes need to relax deeply, often."[97] Make a habit of palming[98] your eyes three times a day to relax and rejuvenate them:

- To palm, simply sit at a desk and place your cupped hands over your closed eyes. (I rub my hands together before palming, to warm them.)
- There should be nothing touching your eyeball; just a warm pocket of air covering them, no pressure.
- Breathe deeply and allow your eyes to rest in the dark space behind your hands – this gives the cells on your retina a much-needed break from close work and tension.
- You'll soon be able to feel how refreshing a few minutes of palming and deep breathing can be!
- When coming out of palming, remove your hands and give your eyes a minute to adjust to the light, then open them and blink 30 times or so.

Eyesight is something we rarely think about until the eyes are not seeing as clearly as before; then the tendency is to go the optician and take whatever glasses he or she suggests. Yet I know from having had glasses in the past that using the eyes in a more considerate way and relaxing them through palming, can improve eyesight. I am older now and don't need glasses.

"Sunning"[99] is another easy and relaxing way to care for your eyes according to Joy Thompson, a Natural Vision educator in British Columbia and Margaret Montgomery, a Bates Method Practitioner in England. According to Joy Thompson, "Our eyes need the stimulation of full-spectrum light, so during the summer months, get out in the morning or late afternoon sunshine without sunglasses and let yourself take the sunshine in! Blink often throughout the day to stimulate your eye muscles and keep your cornea refreshed".[100]

Finally, splashing the eyes can soothe the facial muscles and relax the eyes. This involves splashing the eyes with cold and warm water, morning and night. In the morning, start with warm water and go to cold water to finish. In the evening, start with cold water and finish with warm. I find this very relaxing for the eyes prior to sleep.

MELTing

Back to the rest of the body. Another beneficial self-treatment for the body which, according to Sue Hitzmann creator of MELT, "re-hydrates the connective tissue - the missing link to pain-free living" is the MELT method (MELT).[101] MELT helps prevent pain, heal injury and erase the negative effects of aging and daily living.[102] By using various sized small 100% rubber balls MELT helps the body release long-held tension. Typing this book I have enjoyed the tension relief that using MELT balls brings.

I am astonished at how much more foot and hand flexibility I have. I have not MELTed every day but when I don't I wonder why I haven't, as I feel so much better when I do; but I have noticed that my hands feel like they have more blood flow and I can type faster. (Anecdotal evidence but nice results nonetheless.)

The MELT method tackles the results from daily repetitive movements and postures that cause connective tissue dehydration and, over time, "stuck stress" and inflammation.

MELT is about having a body that's efficient and balanced. It's not intended to just improve flexibility. Some people are hyper-mobile, those people find increased stability in their joints with it. MELT brings balance in the hydration and helps both sides of the spectrum restore the balance in their own body. It's amazing how it works but it really does.[103]

A girl friend of mine who had plantar fasciitis used the MELT balls (she introduced me to them) and no longer suffers from it. (I have listed where to find MELT balls in the Appendix.)

Knowing all these hints and tricks only shows me how unwise we are to spend hours indoors, reading on the Internet or watching television and not moving. Put inactivity alongside our junk food lifestyle[104] and we could well be setting our selves up for disaster.

GIVE IT A GO

- Incorporate movement into your day throughout the day. Sitting still at a desk for seven hours and then flogging yourself in the gym is not very balanced so why not get up and move about every hour and stretch to the ceiling? If you can, go outside for ten deep breaths. The time away from your desk may well bring clarity.
- If you are fortunate to be a stay at home mum or work for yourself, why not get up and go for a walk when the sun comes out? Sunshine is your friend! I find if I am struggling with an article, a brisk walk clears my head and brings inspiration. It brightens my mood too!
- Don't be afraid of moving, roll your shoulders, stick your tongue out whilst at your desk, relax your jaw, wiggle your fingers. You are a river, not a pond!

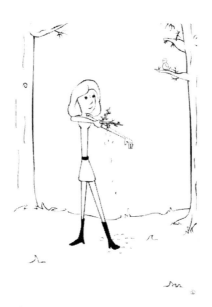

CHAPTER 9

. . .

Get the Rubbish Out!

. . .

Living in the modern world, you very likely come into regular contact with substances, synthetic chemicals and ingredients that are better out of your body than in. If you visit the loo each day you are doing some detoxing but are there other things you can do? Fortunately, yes.

Exercise is important, as we discussed in the last chapter, as it gets the circulation going and stimulates the lymphatic system. The lymphatic system requires muscular movement in order to work or flow. However, many of us have sedentary jobs, sitting at a computer all day and barely moving. That's another good reason to get up and shake and wiggle every half hour. I have spent a long time sitting writing this book but I also have to keep my lymphatic system happy. A healthy lymphatic system is very important.

The lymphatic system is a major part of the body's immune system. It contains "a clear liquid, rich in white blood cells. It flows through us via lymphatic vessels, which are intertwined with our blood vessels."[105] Lymph conveys to the blood the final products of digested food. It also receives from the blood waste products of metabolism. Un-eliminated wastes form cellulite[106] (surprise! Bet you always wanted to know about that!), but "if the lymph is circulating freely is almost impossible to get sick."[107]

Stimulating the Lymphatic System

It is possible to stimulate lymphatic drainage and improve the appearance of the skin.[108] "Body brushing" is a surprisingly simple way to do this (and is thought to assist with improving cellulite). Body brushing only takes a minute and may help to remove toxins from the body.[109] This is a do-it-yourself at home routine that is well worth considering adding into your day. You can find body brushes in most chemists and natural health food stores. When I body brush I wonder why I don't do it more often!

Even if you are taking exercise you are likely not giving yourself a full body massage each day—who has the time for that?

There are some old fashioned preventative measures that may keep your immune system happy and are easy to incorporate into your daily routine. Breast massage is a simple way of keeping the breasts healthy and encouraging sound lymphatic flow.

Going back to the pond and river analogy; one is relatively stagnant and one is flowing. We want the body to flow. Gentle exercise is a good way to accomplish this but so is self-massage. It's easy to do after a shower and this is the sort of prevention I feel needs to be taught in school. Women shouldn't have to live in fear but be empowered with positive ways to look after and care for their precious body.

If, over the years, we use synthetic chemicals, like moisturisers and deodorants, then our bodies have to deal with these. Additionally, if you wear underwired bras you should be sure they are fitted properly and not digging into the breast, which might upset optimum lymphatic flow. I actually rarely wear a bra and when I do it is a non-wired one.

In my teenage years I had a fibrocystic breast lump that was removed. The attending surgeon, who deals with breast cancer, advised me to do two things. I promised I would do them throughout my life:

1. Only wear a bra when absolutely necessary (such as a party where the dress would not look right without one).
2. Relax and de-stress, do gentle exercise and find some form of peaceful exercise I enjoy.

I have not bought an ill-fitting bra since—that was 22 years ago! Breasts obviously differ in size and many women who have large breasts find a bra altogether more comfortable but if you have smaller breasts, consider perhaps having a 'no bra day' once in a while.

Self-massage allows our lymphatic system to 'move along please' any substances that may get stored in the fatty tissue. Good lymphatic drainage can be achieved through this simple routine, which can be done once or twice a week. It is better to do it once a week than not at all.

Lymphatic breast massage is "specifically moving the breast in a way that mimics how lymph moves in the body."[110] According to Lara Koljonen, who also promotes lymphatic breast massage for women in California, "Breast health is movement".[111] I have been doing the Breast Health Project exercises since 2012 and they are very simple, I often do them whilst waiting for the kettle to boil.

Breast Massage

Remember, if you only did the pumping of the armpit, but you did it every time you bathed, you would be improving breast health every day!

Put your hand in your armpit and push inward and upward. Go deep into the armpit. Pump upward and release. Do this ten to twenty times.

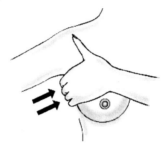

Hold your entire breast and move it upward toward the armpit. If your breasts are large, this may take more than one hand position. Do this ten times.

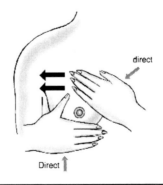

Hold your breast and pump directly inward toward the chest wall. Do this five to ten times.

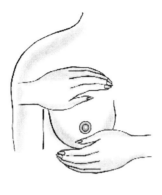

Holding your breast stable, pump the upper inner quadrant of your breast up towards your neck. Do this five to ten times.

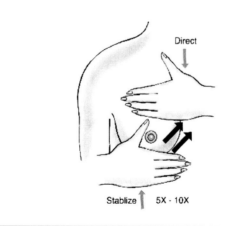

Pictures reproduced by kind permission of Daya Fisch, Director of the BreastHealthProject.com

Hydrotherapy

Another way to stimulate the lymphatic system is by hot and cold showering or hydrotherapy.[112] We are very fortunate that there is a very smart outdoor spa near our home. It has a luxurious, hot sauna, a cool plunge pool and the peaceful silence of resting rooms. But you can recreate this at home too, if you have a shower or bath.

It really is as simple as having a shower, then towards the end turning the temperature to cold—not the coldest—and splashing your body (be brave!). Get under the shower completely for about 10 to 20 seconds. Get out of the shower, dry yourself and, if you have time, rest on your bed for ten minutes, or go about your day. Initially it is very bracing! This hydrotherapy can stimulate blood flow.[113]

Looking radiant requires that the lymphatic system is working optimally!

Sweating

Sweating has an important function in the body, which is to regulate body temperature. Contrary to popular belief sweating has relatively little to do with detoxification and as little as one percent of heavy metals are excreted through sweat, the majority being through urine and faeces.[114] That said, a sauna feels amazing and I'll keep enjoying them!

Antiperspirants are a bizarre invention, in my opinion. Why would I wish to stop a process that is designed to regulate my body temperature by using a substance that keeps things in my body?

I bought into the whole hype in my teenage years and rolled antiperspirant with the best of them. I must have bought bottles of the stuff. No more! I now use nothing and I still have friends—unless they are not telling me something? Hmm.

Deodorant can help deal with the odour of sweat but it isn't going to stop you sweating. We don't want to do that, as that is an important function of the body. Antiperspirants commonly have aluminium (aluminum if you live in America), which is a metal and often mentioned in discussions about Alzheimer's disease. There are enough dubious substances with which we come into contact in our lives, that I am not voluntarily going to pay to put a synthetic chemical and metal solution under my arms. 'Au naturel' is for me. If you want to use a deodorant I have listed a few I have used and liked in the Appendix.

Alternatively, you can make an easy deodorant recipe. I do not take credit for it; it comes from a blog called "How About Orange". I spoke to Jessica and she is happy for me to use it (see Appendix for web address). I then set about playing skin care creator in my kitchen. Feel free to adapt it to suit you. I like this paste, which is easy to massage under the arms and there is no plastic bottle to throw away or recycle. Recipe follows on page 125.

Castor Oil

This is quite an old fashioned remedy but in the last few years I have used it with astonishing results. This year there were a lot of nasty colds, flu and the horrid vomiting bug doing the rounds. Many of our friends succumbed and just before Christmas I felt well below par. I was not ill as such, merely not running at my usual 100 percent. I also found that I had a lump in my breast that directly coincided with where my lymph nodes are.

Obviously, as a woman and with so much media fear surrounding breast cancer, I thought "Ooh that isn't good!" Yet, common sense prevailed: this lump appeared out of nowhere, was very sore and was exactly at the time when all those around me were lying in bed with flu or racing to the bathroom with worse ailments.

As an ever-practical person, I looked in my books and then remembered all about castor oil (not for drinking, before you concern yourself). I use castor oil in a compress over an area of the body in need of attention. Castor oil is an ancient remedy that has been documented as being used to benefit the lymphatic system, assist acne, improve fungal toenails and ease aching muscles and sore joints as well as all manner of other ailments.[115] The University of Maryland Medical Center suggests using a castor oil pack for pelvic inflammatory disease.[116] I have found it works well on ingrown hairs too! Castor oil is also used in some versions of the Oil Cleansing Method with great results.

How to...

Castor Oil Compress

- Buy good quality castor oil. Use an oil washcloth that you do not mind getting oily and sticky. Then you'll need cling film or plastic food wrap, a bin bag, a couple of old towels, a hot water bottle and a bed or sofa on which to relax.
- Warm the oil in a bowl over a pan of water; do not microwave! This is just to make sure it is not too cold on the skin—be sure it is not too hot. Make up a hot water bottle.
- Prepare the area where you will lie down, be that your bed or a sofa; put the plastic bin bag and towel down (to protect). Dip the flannel into the castor oil. Cover the area of your body that requires attention with the castor oil flannel (washcloth); cover with food wrap and another towel. Then place the hot water bottle on the area. Lie down or recline and relax for up to an hour.
- I find a castor oil pack is wonderfully calming and relaxing. I also notice a sense of increased energy in any area that I place a pack. When using a castor oil pack, I usually drift off to sleep.

Laughter

A cheerful disposition is good for your health.
~Proverbs 17:22

According to *Psychology Today*, the average four-year old laughs 300 times a day. Once we get to 40, that figure goes down to a horrifyingly low four times a day![117]

Laugher is the best medicine. It helps to tone your tummy, improve your mood and ease pain, too. In his fascinating book, *Anatomy of an Illness*, Norman Cousins describes how ill he once was and how laughter helped immensely. He decided to watch funny films and laugh whilst lying in bed ill. Laughing, he says, "…worked. I made the joyous discovery that ten minutes of genuine belly laughter had an anesthetic effect and would give me at least two hours of pain-free sleep. When the pain-killing effect of the laughter wore off, we would switch on the motion-picture projector again and not infrequently it would lead to another pain-free sleep interval."[118]

During my Nia Brown Belt I had to spend a minute each day laughing. The first time I did this in a group felt really uncomfortable; I felt self-conscious, nervous and rather silly. The time went really slowly. I still did the minute's laughing but on the last day of the course I realised a minute's laughing seemed to pass faster and I was beginning to enjoy it.

Somehow the more you laugh, the more you can find to laugh about. Laughing can also reduce stress and enhance quality of life. "Virtually all studies of laughter and health indicate positive results."[119] I have found if I am really fed up, a good laugh works wonders.

According to Robert Provine, laughter is for "bringing people together."[120] In an increasingly fragmented society I think we need more laughter, don't you?

Q: Why did the tomato go out with a prune?
A: Because he couldn't find a date!

I hope that made you giggle?

GIVE IT A GO

- Laugh for a minute each day. Initially it may feel odd, you might feel silly or start laughing and feel too uncomfortable. Persevere.
- One of the benefits of the Internet is there are many comedy show snippets you can watch. My favourites are Michael McIntyre, Miranda Hart, The Two Ronnies and Despicable Me. If you don't like British humour you can find many others!
- Smile randomly throughout the day and sense how it feels in your body. It gives you a lift and may encourage you to pass that smile on. They are free to share!

HOW TO MAKE...

Deodorant

INGREDIENTS:
60g tapioca flour or arrowroot powder
60g baking soda
35g coconut oil
5-10 drops of your favourite organic essential oil
150ml small jar with lid

METHOD:
• Mix the flour, baking soda and coconut oil together.
• If the coconut oil is too solid, melt over a pan of simmering water. Once the coconut oil is melting, mix further.
• Add the drops of essential oil—you might be tempted to put in more drops. Start with less or it may be overpowering and itchy on your skin!
• Pour carefully into the pot. You can use any excess in the following days—shame to waste it. Or put it in a sample pot and give to a girlfriend.

(Note: Some may find baking soda causes itchiness; if so, use more arrowroot and less baking soda. This deodorant may stop your armpits smelling but it is not an anti-perspirant.)

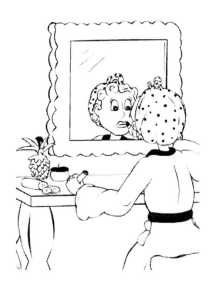

CHAPTER 10

. . .

Edible Skin Care

. . .

When I first learnt that one of the reasons my acne was so bad was in part due to the skin care products I was using, I felt cheated, angry and upset. I had paid for these products and they were not helping.

That said it would be unfair of me to lay blame on skin care products entirely. No one can test for the thousands of combinations we could use on our skin each day. How can they? I can buy brand X cleanser and brand Y lotion—and what do X and Y together create? No one knows! The huge variety of skin care and cosmetic products on the market today gives endless combinations we can create by using many different products each day.

We are the guinea pigs, unless you buy genuinely edible skin care! In the United States the Food and Drug Administration states that "Cosmetic products and ingredients are not subject to FDA pre-market approval authority, with the exception of color additives."[121] In the UK "the manufacturer (or the person responsible for placing the product on the market in the European Community) is primarily responsible for ensuring that cosmetic products do not cause damage to human health when applied under normal or reasonably foreseeable conditions of use."[122] The FDA's website simply says, "Cosmetic firms are responsible for substantiating the safety of their products and ingredients before marketing."[123]

Cosmetics in Canada are subject to the cosmetic notification rule, which means within the first ten days after a product comes to market Health Canada has to be informed.[124] That seems a little worrying considering a lotion containing 'heaven knows what' may be on the market for ten days prior to Health Canada knowing about it.

I truly believe a bridge must be built between real food and real skin care.

. . . .

Skin care must be good enough to eat!

. . . .

If skin care isn't good enough to eat, you may be putting a low dose of synthetic chemicals into your bloodstream through the products you put on your skin.

Trans-dermal patches were developed by pharmaceutical companies and are prescribed by doctors to administer medications through the patient's skin. These patches provide an effective way of absorbing a substance through the skin into the blood stream. Just think for a moment about your body lotion, which also goes onto your skin; do you know what ingredients are in it? Have you ever looked? Do you know if you are rubbing synthetic chemicals onto your skin? Trans-dermal patches and lotions are not dissimilar. If trans-dermal patches work, which they do, then surely we need to be more careful of what is in our lotions and skin care potions? There is scientific evidence that a percentage of some substances is absorbed through the skin![125]

. . . .

Unless you diligently read the labels on your skin care you could be rubbing synthetic chemicals into your skin.

. . . .

That's why it is vital to read labels. Companies can create skin care products using ingredients tested in isolation but very rarely in the for-mulas in which they appear on the shelves. The FDA says "the safety of a product can be adequately substantiated through (a) reliance on already available toxicological test data on individual ingredients and on product formulations that are similar in composition to the particular cosmetic."[126] How similar is similar though? Doesn't that mean a company can make an assumption that if certain ingredients are similar in composition then they must be okay?

The final decision on safety lies with the company producing the product with no independent testing. Just edible skin care for me!

United States Food and Drug Administration researchers detected lead in 400 brands of lipstick.[127] Yet the FDA's authority over cosmet-ics is somewhat limited and restricted to "information that comes to us. We do it by the monitoring of adverse events that come into the FDA." Essentially they look for trends. They keep an eye on reports that come in and gauge if there have been, for example, lots of problems with a shower gel or a body lotion. "If there are certain trends that come through that suggest that there may be a safety issue, it sets off a flag for us to delve a little more fully."[128]

What this means for you as a consumer, is that you may potentially be the guinea pig when using the lipstick, mascara or lotions you buy, unless you read your labels and choose wisely. The precautionary principle is rarely used in the skin care and cosmetics industry. In fact, the opposite often happens: products are only removed when consumers complain.

Perfumes and Scents with a Hidden Secret

Fragrances and perfumes are not as kind a present as many husbands and partners might think; perfume often contains a nasty little secret. If you still wear regular perfume then there is a good chance you are using a product containing phthalates (pronounced THAL-ates), which are synthetic chemicals used in perfumes and, curiously, to soften plastics. You can tell if a product is likely to contain phthalates by looking for "fragrance" or "parfum" on the skin care or cosmetics label.

Phthalates are endocrine disruptors (i.e., the thyroid, adrenals, reproductive system, etc.—a complex system). In February 2013 the United Nations Environment Programme (UNEP) and the World Health Organization (WHO) released a report on the State of the Science of Endocrine Disrupting Chemicals, which outlined the stark reality that our reliance on synthetic chemicals is a "global threat."[129]

According to scientists at Washington University, phthalates could have a negative impact on hormones, potentially bringing on early menopause for some women.[130] These synthetic chemical hormone-mimicking substances[131] are also linked to foetal abnormalities.[132] They can be found in some natural-labelled products too so, once again, reading labels is paramount!

Perfumes can be very strong and some people are sensitive to them; so perhaps we have a responsibility to not wear perfume for others' sake? You likely know that feeling of walking past someone in the street only to be overwhelmed by his or her fragrance? Yes? That synthetic chemical bombardment is so offensive that some companies,[133] councils and universities in some areas now promote scent-free policies.[134] This makes me happy! You smell beautiful without squirting three sprays of "eau du toxic whatnot" on yourself.

. . . .

"Consumers believe that 'if it's on the market, it can't hurt me'.
And this belief is sometimes wrong."[135]
John Bailey, Ph.D

. . . .

Much of modern skin care is not edible; not even remotely! Did you know that the petrolatum in many lip balms is an oil derivative! It was discovered when a man investigating the oil rigs in Pennsylvania in the 1800s found that the "rod wax", that caused the drilling rigs' oil pumps to seize up, was being used by workers on their skin for cuts; it was later marketed as petroleum jelly.[136]

I put petrol (gas to North Americans) in my car; I want to use different substances on my skin. Why would anyone put petrolatum on their lips? Perhaps, the same reason I used to for years, I simply didn't know I had to read ingredient labels.

I just trusted that if it was on the shelf, it must be safe. I am not alone. Relatively few women know that each day they are using a synthetic chemical cocktail on their skin. Some ingredients, when used in an industrial setting, warrant a mask, gloves and the warning, "In case of contact, flush skin with plenty of water."[137] Yet this particular example, propylene glycol, is commonly found in shampoos, moisturisers, shower gels and other products I could use on my skin. It seems incongruous that a skin care product can contain an ingredient that the work place deems unwise to touch! The concentrations might vary widely but when so many genuinely natural alternatives exist I think we are wise to read labels.

The fact that ingredients in some skin care products can be harmful is a guarded secret and one that the multi-billion dollar skincare industry may wish to keep that way. One of the world's largest skin care and cosmetic companies posted profits in excess of two billion US dollars[138] in 2011. With profits like that there might be little incentive to change formulas and cease using synthetic chemicals. After all, women are buying these products willingly and cosmetics houses expect these levels of sales to continue.[139]

So why is there not outrage? Perhaps women simply don't know that reading ingredients labels is necessary. I didn't for years. I just liked the pictures and image that was associated with the products. John E. Bailey, Ph.D. and former director of the office of cosmetics and colors at the FDA has said, "Image is what the cosmetic industry sells through its products and it's up to the consumer to believe it or not."[140]

TV advertising is especially expensive and any company that can afford such advertising is invariably earning a considerable amount. Many advertised products are produced with one goal in mind; to create brand awareness and sell lots of product units. The adverts I have seen usually play on your self-esteem to pitch the merits of transformative cosmetics.

What about 'Organic'?

I would argue that even the term "organic" these days is not so much about natural skin care as it is about marketing. Products may have pretty labels, claims and nice looking boxes but "organic" can be used on products with very few truly organic ingredients.[141] "The term 'organic' is not defined in either of these laws or the regulations that FDA enforces under their authority."[142]

It is really only if a product has the USDA organic logo that there is any real guarantee of all organic ingredients; if a product carries the USDA logo then it must consist of 95 percent organic ingredients. "Made with organic ingredients" has to consist of at least 70 percent organic ingredients. Yet a product can say "organic ingredients" and be less than 70 percent of organic origin.[143] So you can see how very confusing it is! That is why reading labels is so important.

A certified organic product (by the USDA in the U.S.A., Soil Association in the UK or COSMos in Europe) is often a guarantee of what you are buying. Eco Cert requires just five to ten percent organic ingredients to be able to display the Eco Cert certification, meaning 95 percent of the ingredients might not be certified organic. It is wise to check certification standards in your region.

Companies wishing profit from the growing demand for organic skin care and cosmetics can make appealing-sounding claims on their labels, knowing that customers are seeking organic and natural products. The flip side of this, is that a growing number of companies are removing endocrine disrupting chemicals like parabens and claiming that as a benefit on their labels.[144] What do they replace parabens with? That's why I like to use edible ingredients and keep it simple!

"Natural" is another over-used word in the skin care industry. Natural doesn't necessarily mean what you'd associate with nature. There is no legal definition of what natural is. Cosmetics are governed by no specific regulations about added value labelling or advertising claims.[145] Companies can use "natural", or "clean", "pure" and "nourishing" as marketing buzz-words or even in the name of their company but a quick read of the ingredients may tell a different story.

"Paraben-free" is a label that is often used on cosmetics today but this can simply mean another preservative (about which we know even less) has been used instead.

"Green washing" is when a product label features flowers, leaves or cucumbers, for example, and appealing words to give the illusion that the product is "natural", "organic", "green" or "eco-friendly" to achieve a competitive advantage. It is rife within the skin care industry and the household cleaning industry.

Cosmetic Consequences

You likely know about the concept of a "carbon footprint", which is linked to how much you drive, fly or burn fossil fuels to heat your home. Have you ever thought about the environmental impact of the *cosmetics* you buy? What does the list of ingredients actually mean and what happens to them when they get washed down the drain? All our choices have an *impact* either on us, or those around us, as well as others further afield. Change can be challenging but sometimes it is very necessary for our own sake and for the sake of others.

A "Cosmetic Footprint" labeling system is something I would like to see on skin care and cosmetics products. This would be a grading system considering product ingredients and the resulting impact "downstream", as Sandra Steingraber says."[146] Perhaps a 1-10 scale for safety; one for safe and edible and 10 for harmful!

Maybe you think, "Well, I can't worry about everything". Yes; that is futile. Action, however, is more successful. I am encouraging you to consider the impact of your personal care choices on our health, water supply and our wider environment.

There are, for example, tiny plastic beads in some shower gels and exfoliating soap products that get washed down the drain[147] resulting in fish thinking, "Ooh, yummy food", which of course it isn't. Unfortunately water treatment plants can't remove them as they're too small. Fortunately some companies are phasing polyethylene microbeads out[148] but for the others that aren't – read labels!

. . . .

Consider the impact of your personal care choices on our health, water supply and our wider environment.

. . . .

Perfumes are not simply an issue for humans, yet again our personal care choices affect others further afield. According to a 2004 Stanford University study, the endocrine disrupting phthalates (dibutyl phthalate) in household fragrances might be harming aquatic wildlife.[149]

Even if we accept that humans have a choice, what about those life forms, that are "living downstream" from us?[150] Animals and fish that live in the sea don't have any choice but to live with the effects.[151] At the very least we can filter the water we drink. What you use gets washed down the drain; do you ever think about that whilst buying shampoo or cosmetics?

I never used to think about what I was buying and certainly not about my cosmetic footprint. Now I mainly make my own skin care or only buy from companies that really care about what goes into their products. I can't rely on what a label says. I now know *I have to read ingredients carefully, each and every time I shop!*

Lessen Your Cosmetic Footprint

I encourage you to make non-toxic personal care choices. My list of questionable ingredients are:

- **Triclosan** - antibacterial products often contain triclosan.
- **Sodium lauryl sulphate** (spelt sulfate in North America) or sodium laureth sulphate – found in shampoo, toothpaste and shower gel.
- **Fragrance or parfum, perfume** - watch out for unfragranced products as they can still have a masking fragrance – check the labels, you'll often see it!
- **Parabens** - methyl, ethyl, butyl, isopropyl and benzyl are all preservatives.
- **Cyclomethicone, dimethicone and cyclopentasiloxane** - silicone, very common in moisturisers and conditioners.
- **Sodium hydroxymethylglycinate, DMDM hydantoin, imidazolidinyl urea and Quaternium-15** - formaldehyde releasing agents.
- **Dibutyl phthalate** - is often found in nail polish.
- **Petrolatum** - is petroleum jelly.
- **Diethanolamine (DEA), polyethylene glycol (PEG)**
- **Polyethylene, polyethylene microspheres**

The following tips will reduce your cosmetic footprint (and detox your bathroom) in seven *simple* steps. Set the timer for twenty minutes and do what you can in that time. It is less daunting that way!

1. **Out with the OLD!** Look at the Period After Opening (PAO) symbol and throw away anything that you know has been open longer than recommended. (When you buy new products, use a marker pen to write on the product when you bought it!)

2. **Read labels** and put in a bin anything that has "parfum" or "fragrance" on the label. According to Rick Smith, "parfum" and "fragrance" are "hide-all" words.[152] "Parfum" can actually hide hundreds of different synthetic chemicals that do not have to be listed on the label.[153] What that means is that endocrine disrupting phthalates can be hiding in products labeled "parfum" or "fragrance". You don't want them on your skin or in your body. (Phthalates are also thought to be obesogens.[154])

3. **Look at your shampoo and liquid soaps.** If they contains sodium lauryl sulphate, then add that to the bin too. SLS, as it is also known, is thought to be a skin sensitiser.[155]

4. **Throw away air fresheners** unless they are essential oils. Air fresheners contain an array of ingredients[156] such as phthalates, which as you know by now are likely detrimental to our health.[157] They may actually exacerbate indoor air pollution via the addition of toxic chemicals to the atmosphere.[158]

5. **Love bacteria**—don't antibacterial yourself! Antibacterial products often contain triclosan, which is thought to be an endocrine disruptor and contribute to antibacterial resistance.[159] I think antibacterial products are irresponsible as triclosan can end up in the water and soil.[160]

6. **Use vinegar** and essential oils instead of regular cleaners containing synthetic chemicals which get washed down the drain. Use the household products database from the U.S. Department of Health and Human Services.[161] This lists ingredients and enables you to find out what is *really* in your cleaning products!

7. **Clean your bathroom** with simple ingredients like baking soda and Castile soap or Miessence's Bio Pure which is probiotic and

industrial strength but non-toxic. (See Appendix.) Remember, what you wash down the drain (shampoo, toothpaste, antibacterial soap or hair dye) ends up in someone else's water!

The planet is a cycle (remember the pictures of clouds, rain and rivers from geography class in your childhood?). Surely each one of us has a responsibility to not pollute? Whilst you are in detoxing mode, why not consider your household-chemical footprint too? Household cleansers do not list the full ingredients very often so you can buy products without knowing what is in them. Claims like "98% natural", "60% plants-based" and "supporting the environment" are misleading and dubious. I have even seen an antibacterial washing up liquid (dish soap) that claimed to be supporting the environment. As Adria Vasil says "there is a tsunami of greenwashing."[162]

Cosmetic Clutter

Just because there is a myriad of personal care products available doesn't mean you have to buy them. I wonder how much you'd save each year if you simplified your skin care and household cleaning regime? Seven years ago I detoxed my bathroom and now I use very few products (I will discuss this in a moment). I love using less products and having less *cosmetic clutter*. I have saved hundreds of dollars, my skin looks better, and I can walk past a department store with a skin care special offer and smile knowing I don't have to buy it.

. . . .

Skin care simplicity is freedom!

. . . .

I like ingredients like jojoba oil; you can actually cleanse your face with it. It has good compatibility with the skin's natural sebum[163] as any of the oils on the market. Jojoba oil contains antioxidants and is easily absorbed into the skin.

It's important to realise that the skin actually can look after itself. Otherwise how did women survive before we had department stores with their many skin care products? The Romans used to use olive oil to cleanse. Olive oil is even recommended in the Bible for skin care: "… olive oil to soothe their skin" (Psalm 104:15).

I have family friends, ladies in their 80s and 90s, who all said they never use soap on their skin. They only ever use a flannel and occasionally some genuinely natural moisturiser. It seems that simplicity is the best kept beauty secret.

Embracing Natural Beauty

Regardless of what the advertising claims, you do not need dozens of products to make you look beautiful. You are beautiful already. Say "I am beautiful". You really are. However, it can feel nice to have a relaxing facial or massage; just be aware of what you are using. Many perceived high end organic companies purport to be natural and professional but still use many synthetic chemical ingredients and petroleum derivatives. Why would you want to put that on your skin and pay for the privilege?

Also remember that price is little indicator of quality and heavily advertised products might not be what they seem. For years I wanted the latest cream I saw advertised. I especially liked "limited edition" products which I bought as I didn't want to miss out (which I now know was just clever marketing, using the scarcity technique[164]).

I never stopped to look at the ingredients' list; I just wanted to look beautiful. My thoughts were on what the product would transform me into, not investigating the finer details of ingredients like propylene glycol, dimethicone, parabens and butylene glycol. I paid hundreds of pounds at beauty salons for facials and was told, 'This product will really help with your acne-ridden skin'. In my desperation for clear skin, I bought it, yet a few days later I would have a rash or itchy skin until I stopped using it. My skin felt better when I did not use such products!

Thankfully there are some great products on the market and today, more than ever, there are ethical companies providing sound, organically grown products that really work. Oil cleansing is gaining in popularity which isn't as scary as it sounds (to a former acne sufferer anything oil is horrifying).

Oil Cleansing

I now use the oil cleansing method (OCM). I started using Helena Lane's Oil Cleanser, locally made in Vancouver. Her cleanser is simplicity itself, made from jojoba oil, beeswax and lavender essential oil. Pretty simple! It felt weird initially but now I have skin that is low maintenance and I get lots of compliments on my great-looking skin.

You have to get over the fear of oil. I can't do that for you. It is gaining acceptance but is still not mainstream so you may be on your own on this one. What I really like about oil cleansing is that I cleanse at night and then don't have to do anything, none of the fuss of serums, toner this and that. My skin breathes at night and I wake up with "normal" looking skin—not oily or dry, just healthy looking skin. For its simplicity alone oil cleansing is certainly something to consider.

There are many other companies that make oil cleansers; ones I have tried and like are The Organic Pharmacy Carrot Butter Cleanser, Neal's Yard Remedies Wild Rose Beauty Balm and Helena Lane's Lavender and Lime Cleanser. Alternatively you can actually make your own oil cleansing base. There are two options, one with castor oil and one without.

The OCM uses a blend of castor oil and either jojoba, olive or sunflower oil to gently cleanse the face. I was sceptical as castor oil is very sticky. Initially I disregarded the whole OCM idea, thinking I have far better things to do with my time, but I was curious and tried it. I found it is inexpensive and works!

The fun of making your own skin care product is that you can personalise it to whatever oil you feel like.

HOW TO MAKE...

Castor Oil Cleanser

INGREDIENTS:
Castor oil
Sunflower oil or jojoba oil (organic if you prefer)
100mls bottle: brand new with a pump
Organic essential oil

METHOD:

For oily skin:
- 30 mls of castor oil to 70 mls sunflower oil

For balanced skin:
- 20 mls castor oil to 80 mls sunflower oil

For dry skin:
- 10 mls castor oil to 90 mls sunflower oil

10 drops (literally) of essential oil. I like lavender at the moment but have used lemon and also orange. You choose!

Oil & Beeswax Cleanser

I make a cleanser of jojoba oil and beeswax. I include some essential oil but that isn't necessary and if you have sensitive skin omit it. Ideally use an organic essential oil.

INGREDIENTS:
An 80ml glass pot with a lid to store your fabulous finished cleanser
A new / clean chopstick
A double boiler or little saucepan with a heatproof bowl that fits in the top but doesn't touch the bottom of the pan
60mls jojoba oil
11g beeswax - preferably organic or from a local source

METHOD:
Accurately measure the oil and beeswax, put into the glass bowl and gently melt over simmering water in a saucepan. Use a clean chopstick to stir the mixture until melted. When cooling, add seven drops of lavender essential oil. (Less is more with the oils, they are concentrated plant oils!) Gently pour your cleanser into the glass storage jar. Gently tap the jar on the bottom to bring any bubbles to the top. Put the lid on and store in a cool, dark place.

<u>How to cleanse your face at night:</u>

Put a small amount of cleanser on your face and gently massage into the skin for a minute or two. Pay attention to the nose and any areas where you might have blackheads. Either remove straight away or leave for a few minutes. Run a clean basin of warm water and use the flannel to remove the cleanser, rinsing regularly. You may need to repeat if you wear lots of make up and foundation.

This nourishing cleanser removes the day's dirt and grime and is moisturising enough to prevent the skin drying out. At night I do not use anything else after cleansing—the aim is to cleanse the skin and let it breathe. Lovely and simple, isn't it?

<u>Morning skin care:</u>

I use a clean flannel in a clean basin of warm water to refresh my face. I then do "splashing", which not only helps my skin but refreshes my eyes. I half fill a basin with warm water and then turn on the cold tap (gently) and splash my face until the water is quite cold. This refreshes my eyes and I'm ready to face the day. In winter I might use a pea-sized amount of aloe vera (inner-leaf gel), in summer I'll spritz flower water followed by a drop of rose hip oil or dab of shea butter.

See? Skin care can be wonderfully simple. It is important to note how your skin feels and start to tune in to how it changes on a daily basis! This skin awareness will tell you a lot; what foods suit you, how much water to drink and how much sleep is necessary. The body tells us a lot if we only tune in to it.

For numerous other recipes I really like *Cook, Brew and Blend Your Own Herbs* and *Make your Own Cosmetics* by Neal's Yard Remedies. Even though there are many recipes in these books I truly don't think we need them all even if they are home-made! I am sure your local library will have other books too.

Baths

Baths are a traditional way of relaxing and easing away the day's stresses and worries, soothing the body, mind and spirit. The city of Bath, in England, has therapeutic baths and years ago people would gather and socialise at the baths, taking in the therapeutic minerals of the area.

Mineral salts are beneficial in many ways. When the body is stressed, it can benefit from magnesium[165] and other trace minerals. You can recreate this old-fashioned bath experience at home with a warm bath, soft lighting and peace and quiet. It allows me to gain perspective on life and relax.

Many swear by a bath with Epsom salts (rich in magnesium) as a way to soothe the body. I use Epsom salts after a long, cold day skiing. I find the magnesium is nothing short of miraculous. Epsom salts can also be beneficial if you have aching muscles. So, before you reach for the painkillers, why not sink into an Epsom salt bath first? I have a glass of water before I bathe as a hot bath makes me thirsty.

A herbal bath is another way to revive a tired mind after a long day. A muslin bag of a teaspoon with lavender flowers can be calming. Once you have used the bag you can hang it up to dry and use it again.

I also like to add oats to a bath in a little muslin bag. Oats are very soothing for the skin and are thought to assist with eczema. I have used an oats soak on my skin when I have had a very sore rash on my feet; it worked brilliantly. A cup of oats in a washing up bowl with warm water is a soothing soak.

Don't Over Do It

One of the things about our modern skin care consumerism is the is tendency to over wash. All the beauty products available—soaps, exfoliators, shower gels, shampoos, cleansers and scrubs—lead us to think we need to slather them on daily. I really do not believe we need to wash as much as most of us do. A shower and washing the hair every day are simply not necessary unless you are a fitness teacher or working outside and getting really muddy. Most of us who work inside the home or have a somewhat sedentary life are simply not getting dirty enough to warrant daily washing.

Obviously there is a fine line between over washing and not washing enough but if you do the 'sniff test' and your armpits are not smelly, then perhaps you can just use a flannel or washcloth and refrain from the shower? I am not suggesting we become a nation of soap dodgers, far from it, but I do think we wash too much!

The hair may well get oilier the more you wash, just like the skin. If you wash it daily and strip the oils, which is what many shampoos do, then the scalp will create its own oil in order to compensate. (The body is very clever with all of its compensatory processes.) When I was at boarding school I was only allowed to wash my hair once a week. I was not used to washing it more often and therefore the hair regulated itself and looked shiny and clean. If I wash it too often, then it starts becoming oily between washes. So, as potentially scary as it may seem to wash your hair less often, that is the answer to having the hair self-regulate. It is a money-saving tip for buying less shampoo!

Some shampoos are quite harsh. Many contain sodium lauryl sulphate (SLS). You might say, "But SLS is in my baby shampoo!" Yes, it is! Just because it says "baby", on the label doesn't mean it is necessarily gentle! If you (or your children) have trouble with itchy or scratchy skin be sure to look at your shampoo or shower gel labels. I like to choose products without sodium lauryl sulphate, I don't think we need to use synthetic chemicals when good alternatives exist. I use a locally-made simple soap, with olive oil and coconut oil (see Appendix for soap options).

On a recent flight to London, a cabin steward had terrible dermatitis on her hands. We were chatting (it's a long way from Vancouver!) and I said that if she was using the soap in the plane's bathroom (which contained sodium lauryl sulphate, triclosan and many other synthetic ingredients) then it might be wise to stop using it and see what happens to the dermatitis. She had only been working with the airline for a few months and the dermatitis began shortly afterwards! I long to find out what became of her but I can only hope she is either on a flight I take so I can ask but above all I hope she finds her painful, itchy hands much improved.

How many of the skin conditions we suffer from are due to the products we are using? I am not laying blame merely asking. If you have any skin care issues then perhaps start using truly simple skin care (less is more) and see how things go.

Learn to Love Clay

I love putting on a clay mask. I find mud is detoxifying for my skin and well as being rejuvenating and toning. A clay mask makes my skin feel tighter. Having rinsed it off and given my face a good massage with some jojoba oil, my skin looks youthful and radiant, seriously!

You don't need to have a facial to enjoy a clay mask. Following are some tips for using mud on your face at home:

- Mix two teaspoons of clay with water using a plastic spoon.
- Apply the mask. Lie on the sofa or bed, put your feet up and relax. Take ten minutes out. Rest.
- Choose a flannel that is not the brand new cream one that matches your bathroom as it **will** get dirty!

- Cover your face with a flannel and allow the mask to absorb the water. Don't scrub away at your face to remove it; gently use a very wet cloth to remove the clay.
- Follow with a cold water splash.
- Massage the skin for a couple of minutes. You don't have to be a massage therapist, you just need to enjoy a soothing massage.
- Nurture your skin. Don't be critical and start noticing the laughter lines; set all that aside.
- Remember, magazines photos are airbrushed—so relax!
- Enjoy it. This is a time to care for you. Radiant women look after their skin. Enjoying a clay mask is a great opportunity for 'me' time.

You may notice that your pores look more refined; some say a clay mask can help reduce blackheads[166] and generally improve the circulation in your skin, depending on what clay you use. There is green clay, pink clay and white clay as well as many other colours with varying properties such as drawing, rejuvenating, re-mineralising, etc. I have a few clay masks and use them depending on how my skin feels. If I have a few spots then I use green clay: I use it daily for two weeks, to get the skin really waking up. (Having had acne for over ten years, I can't believe I did not come across this simple technique earlier). If I want to tone my skin but it feels dry I use a white clay (also known as Kaolin clay, which is the most gentle and least drawing of all the clays). Rhassoul clay is another type of clay used in many high-end face masks.

Bentonite clay is a true multi-use product that allows you to easily assist natural healing in your home. Clay can be used to put on bruises, cuts, abrasions and insect bites.[167] Clay masks can be good on bee stings and also if you have a splinter.[168] I had a splinter in my thumb that I put some mask on and it really helped to draw it out. It didn't magically pop out, obviously, but definitely helped speed the process.

I also use clay on my hair to clean it. It is inexpensive and easy but very messy! I mix bentonite clay and filtered water into a paste. I put this paste on the hair as a 'shampoo' but it obviously doesn't foam! You can also buy ready-made clay paste shampoos (see the Appendix for details).

More Mask Ideas

As Sophie Uliano suggests, in her book *Do It Gorgeously*, camu camu powder is very high in vitamin C. She mixes a capsule of camu camu into her face cream. I actually like to mix a camu camu powder capsule with a little tamanu nut oil or argan oil and use it as a vitamin-C-rich face mask (see Appendix for tamanu nut oil).

Other masks I like are Helena Lane's Clay and White Willow Mask, which contains salix alba; this is antibacterial and astringent. Helena says that the beta-hydroxy acid helps to improve cell renewal and brighten the skin. Certainly since I have been using the clay and white willow mask my skin does look fresh. I vary what I use on my skin. The variety of edible plant oils available means there is something to suit everyone.

Another superb ready-made mask is La Bella Figura Beauty's Bio Active Purifying Mask. This also has white willow as well as honey and a beautiful combination of essential oils, spices and plant oils.

I make an edible face mask with strawberries and oats. The strawberries contain vitamin C and alpha hydroxy acids, which are thought to brighten and exfoliate the skin. These acids are also found in sour milk (lactic acid) and citrus fruits (citric acid), so you could use lemon on the face too—sour milk doesn't appeal to me!

How to Make...

Strawberry Face Mask

INGREDIENTS:

30g local and /or organic strawberries

1 tbsp local honey

1 tbsp porridge oats (oatmeal), crushed very finely

METHOD:

Mix the ingredients into a smooth paste with a blender—a fork works too. If runny, add more crushed oats; if too thick, add another crushed strawberry.

I use this just like any other face mask—relax for ten minutes, remove with a washcloth and warm water. Follow by splashing with cool water. Then apply moisturiser.

And finally, if you want to try something completely different, what about ...

Let Your Hair Go Grey!

"What?" You might be thinking; has Joanna gone bananas? No, it's all good here but for a moment roughly calculate how much you spend a year on having your hair treated. Three hundred pounds, five hundred dollars, a thousand, perhaps you spend fifteen hundred dollars or more? It is not a cheap process.

I don't dye my hair so I had to ask women how much they spend. I discovered one lady spends $2700 a year on having highlights and colour to hide her grey hair. Yet, she was not overly sure what started her doing it. She has to have her hair cut every five weeks and coloured at the same time; that is a lot of synthetic chemicals to which she is being exposed.

Why are we so fearful of grey hair? My hair has a few grey hairs but I have decided to accept them. I would rather spend the money on something else. Many women simply do not have spare money to splash out on hair colour.

The condition of the hair and cut is the part that is noticeable; I am not sure it is the colour. Some of the most beautiful women I know, and celebrities who look stunning, actually do not dye their hair. They are aging gracefully.

My mother, who is very beautiful (I'm biased perhaps), has never dyed her hair, nor has my grandmother or sister. I grew up in a family where you age gracefully, whatever that brings. I guess that is the norm for me, so I just accept it.

Perhaps you think this is simply an extraordinary idea. Yet, if none of us dyed our hair, we'd all look similar and there would be less competition. One of my favourite books, written in 1932, is *The New Home Encyclopedia*. It says, "When a woman is past middle age and her hair is turning grey, she may as well accept the inevitable with good humour and grow old gracefully". I could not agree more. I would add enjoy every day to the full, so that when you do go grey you can say "I enjoyed each day, now I accept myself as I am today".

Many people turn to dyeing their own hair but that is not overly wise as hair dyes contain some harsh synthetic chemicals. In 2012 a British woman died after applying a do-it-yourself hair dye kit to her hair; an allergic reaction led to her death.[169] I truthfully do not think, with all the other pollution in the world that we can't control, we need to be adding yet more synthetic chemicals to our body and the ecosystem. Remember that just because it is on the shelf does not mean you have to buy it.

Often women ask me, "Well, what would you use instead; what are safe alternatives?" My answer is "Don't dye your hair, you will get used to it."

Here's a point to consider: *The Message* bible says in Proverbs 16:31, "Grey hair is a mark of distinction, the award for a God-loyal life".

Who says your hair has to be blonde, brown or black all your life? What about celebrating the fact that you are no longer 21 but have years of wisdom with the odd grey hair here and there? That is what I am doing. Will you join me?

Natural Hair Care

Good advice from the 1930s is, "Many women with beautiful hair always rub olive oil well into the roots of the hair as this helps to open the pores and loosen the dirt in the same way that that oil will help to cleanse the face".[170] Here are some other practical ways to treat your hair naturally:

Brush your hair daily to maintain circulation to the scalp. A head massage feels great and can ease tension. When I brush my hair I feel—and look—better.

Use a natural hair tonic. The herb **rosemary** has been used as a hair tonic for years. Put some leaves in a cup of hot water. Once it has cooled, pour it over your hair. Gently massage into the hair and scalp for a stimulating rinse.

Got dandruff? According to Bruce Fife, using coconut oil on the hair as a conditioner can help to control dandruff.[171] Massage into the hair and scalp; leave in for 15 minutes to a couple of hours. Wash out with a gentle shampoo (see Appendix for shampoo ideas).

Hand Care

You can tell a woman's age by her hands, or so the saying goes. I must admit I have hands that do not look 20 any more. However with some edible substances like shea butter, jojoba oil and peach kernel oil you can have nourished soft hands and look every bit as glamorous as a 20-year old.

Looking after your cuticles with regular moisturising is wise. I use rubber gloves for washing up (most of the time!) and that protects my hands from the harsh surfactants in the washing up (dish washing) liquid. As a chef, I love cooking and with that comes washing up. Gloves are your hands' friends.

Shea butter (or coconut oil) is exceptionally moisturising and I rub it into my nails and hands before bed. I find that moisturising my hands stops chapping and the cuticles are less likely to get dry which is when the temptation to peel them becomes great! That is not a good idea, as I am sure you know.

How to Make...

Nourishing Nail Oil

INGREDIENTS:
50mls dropper bottle
40mls jojoba oil; sunflower oil, safflower or sesame works too!
5 drops of organic lemon essential oil
1 Vitamin E capsule

METHOD:
Put the oil in the bottle, add the essential oils and contents of the Vitamin E capsule. Put the lid on and give a good shake.

Why buy fabulously expensive oils when you can easily make your own!

The key with any nail oil is using it! Regardless of the price, the oil only works if you rub it in three times a day. The act of rubbing my fingers and hands is how I like to increase circulation and improve my nails. Use within a month or two.

Foot oil or balm:
You can even use the same oil on your feet. I use almond oil on my feet for a foot massage, but sunflower oil or sesame oil works too. Setting aside time to rub the oil into your feet is often the trickiest part!

You can also use coconut oil, which is naturally antimicrobial, antifungal and antibacterial. Many people have fungal issues with their feet: athlete's foot, fungal toes nails and general poor condition. Coconut oil is moisturizing and has beneficial properties. You learnt about castor oil for fungal toe nails earlier.

How to Make...

Coconut Foot Oil

INGREDIENTS:
50g jar
40g coconut oil
1 tsp castor oil
4 drops of organic lemon essential oil
1 Vitamin E capsule

METHOD:
Mix all the ingredients together with a clean chop stick. Put in the jar. Tea tree and manuka are great for fungal issues and good for athlete's foot, muscular pain, ringworm and skin infections. Store in a cool, dark place.

You may or may not like the smell of manuka and / or tea tree. If you do not like the smell, consider other anti fungal essential oils such as lavender or eucalyptus. Essential oils, despite being sold in many outlets, are very powerful and must be used wisely and considerately.

Dental Care

Just as many shower gels contain sodium laureth sulphate, so do many toothpastes. I was using a well-known brand for over twenty years, throughout which time I suffered from regular bouts of mouth ulcers (canker sores) and no amount of jazzy ulcer gel helped. It was only after my great-aunt told me about sodium lauryl sulphate that I started to put two and two together and stopped using the toothpaste. I started using a genuinely natural, SLS-free toothpaste. I have not had ulcers since.

So what toothpaste is best to use? Obviously that depends on what you like, but currently I'm using *Earthpaste*, which is simply clay and water with a little bit of essential oils. It is made by Redmond Trading, based in Utah, U.S.A. The paste is easy to use and my teeth certainly look nice and white. Other toothpastes that I have used in the past and likely will use again (variety being the spice of life) are:

Miessence make three toothpastes in mint, lemon and anise flavours, they are flavoured with essential oils. The paste is predominantly aloe vera, which can be very soothing on the gums, as well as good for cleaning the teeth.[175] I also like Miessence's mouthwash, which contains aloe vera and essential oils. Aloe vera is thought to be effective in helping fight germs and cavities.[176]

OraWellness Tooth Oil is another non-toxic toothpaste option, although it is not really a paste! It is almond oil and essential oils, such as manuka, peppermint and spearmint. It's strong and one drop is enough. I hadn't used an oil until I tried this but I liked it. OraWellness encourages you to take an alternative view of your teeth and oral health. They are fans of the Bass brushing method, which is more effective than regular brushing.[177] The Bass method is a gentle way to brush and prevents over brushing and gum damage (quite easy with the exceptionally high-tech, space-age looking brushes today). I used to have receding gums in a couple of places; since using a Bass toothbrush my gums are completely healed.

Give It a Go

- Brush your teeth gently; consider watching the OraWellness videos to learn why gentle brushing is wise.
- Check your toothpaste label: does it have a poison control number? Does it contain triclosan? Perhaps your toothpaste has sodium lauryl sulphate? Do you get ulcers (canker sores)? If so, perhaps consider using a different toothpaste.
- Tally up how much you spend on dying your hair, if you do. Is it a lot?
- If you are feeling creative why not make your own nail oil? Remember using it is what helps your nails!

CHAPTER 11

. . .

Radiance in the Home

. . .

Many modern North American homes are hermetically sealed relying on air conditioning and the age old practice of opening our windows is, for some, outdated. Certainly the freezing cold British Columbian winters do little to encourage throwing open a window. However, fresh air circulation is very important and vital to create a healthy home atmosphere and set us up for radiance.

The temperature of your home is also important. We keep our home at about 17C (62F) and when we light a fire it gets up to a roasting 20C (68F) but I know we are not the norm. Most houses today are very much hotter than they used to be in the past. I find myself having to remove clothing layers if I visit someone's house, where they are sitting in t-shirts. In my own home I prefer to put on a jumper (sweater) and not feel too hot, probably as I grew up in an old house in England and it was never very warm in winter. "Put on a jumper or run up and down the stairs if you are cold", my mother would say. I still do this today; it keeps me fit and warm! A nice aside is that our heating bills are minimal and we rarely get colds.

· 157 ·

As unappealing as it might seem, sleeping in a bedroom with the window open at night, in winter, is actually wise for the fresh air circulation benefits. You may find you sleep better—we do, after all, need oxygen!

Improve Your Indoor Air Quality

If you are using traditional washing powder (laundry liquid), dryer sheets, air fresheners,[178] regular washing up liquid (dish soap) and so on then you are coming into contact with many synthetic chemicals each day. If you are not opening windows then, whilst you are in the house, you are breathing some into your lungs. Dryer sheets and air fresheners contain fragrances and phthalates. The material safety data sheets (MSDS) for some air fresheners show that there is potential toxicity. Yet not all ingredients appear on the box. No law in the U.S.A. requires disclosure of all chemical ingredients in consumer products or in fragrances.[179]

One company's laundry liquid, which is designed with a strong perfume that lingers on the clothes, actually states in their MSDS, "Skin contact: prolonged contact may cause mild, transient irritation". This is somewhat concerning since I do wear my clothes for a prolonged period of time in contact with my skin (don't you?).

Air fresheners

Fragrance ingredients are common in today's consumer products but we are wise to be cautious. Studies of endocrine disruptors and asthma associated chemicals in consumer products found that the highest amount of phthalates were in highly perfumed products.[180] What concerns me about these studies is that the detected chemicals were not listed on the product label.

In years gone by it was soot and ash from an open fire that we had to contend with in the air; now we have the effects of an aerosol can, aromatic candle or highly fragranced shampoo. We have discussed *parfum* in skin care but many hundreds of household products also have artificial fragrances.

Many artificial fragrances are derived from petroleum and contain volatile organic compounds (VOCs). Air fresheners are an example of this and are a billion dollar market but I am not sure they have made our life better. It's strange that the labels clearly state "First aid precautions on inhalation: Remove to fresh air."[181] So this is a product that is called an "air freshener" yet if I spray it and inhale (which I do as I breathe in my home) I'm advised to remove to "fresh air". How silly and unnecessary! Why would I voluntarily buy a can and spray it, or use a contraption to put in the wall that intermittently squirts artificial smells throughout the day? I unplug them if I see them!

There is a great deal of marketing and advertising to persuade you that you are not cleaning the house well enough if it doesn't smell like fields of Provence lavender.

Another line of products that has grown in popularity (judging by the sheer number of shops that have them on sale) is fragranced candles. Candles for the sitting room, kitchen candles and candles to create atmosphere; the only atmosphere I can imagine they would create is one that I would wish to leave!

Plants are a healthy alternative for a number of reasons. If you do not have plants in your house then maybe get some. They are a welcome addition to any home, not least because they look nice and help clean the air.[182] Kentia palms and peace lilies have been found to be effective removers of VOCs, benzene and *n*-hexane.[183] They even keep cleaning the air at night, when there is no light![184] According to the United States Environmental Protection Agency, VOCs are found in: paints, flooring, paint strippers, cleaning supplies, aerosol sprays, disinfectants, moth repellents and air fresheners;[185] which seems crazy as many use them to '*clean*' the air! VOCs are linked to eye, nose and throat irritation, headaches, loss of coordination, nausea and damage to the liver, kidney and central nervous system.[186] They are best avoided then!

Cleaning Your Home Naturally

Another substance in cleaning supplies (other than VOCs) is triclosan and you'll learn about that in a moment. Suffice to say you can clean your house effectively and safely without buying cleaning products that have poison control numbers and undisclosed ingredients.

If you wish to deodorise an area or make a non-toxic air freshener then baking soda is remarkably effective. I have used it for over seven years now and find even the smelliest loo can be transformed. Baking soda in North America comes in dinky little boxes designed for deodorising a fridge. You can use that box but I think pouring a little baking soda into a pretty bowl looks nicer.

How to Make...

Air Freshening Powder

INGREDIENTS:
1 pretty small bowl or ramekin
50g baking soda
5 drops of pure essential oil of your choice

Baking soda is also highly effective for cleaning. I make my own all-purpose cleaner (recipe coming up). It is inexpensive, easy to make and the non-toxic bonus means no synthetic chemicals in our house.

A common fear is that natural cleaning products don't work as well. I can assure you that isn't true today (I have put some product suggestions in the Appendix). I have a clean home and mainly use baking soda, Castile soap and vinegar, although not mixed together.

If used in an industrial setting, many cleaning product ingredients would require a mask, gloves and protective gear according to the material safety data sheets (MSDS). If you don't believe me check the Internet for the MSDS sheet for your brand of cleaner - it's there.

Have you ever looked at the printed warnings? Some are fairly direct: poison warnings, dangers of ingestion and skin contact advice abound. If you are cleaning your home with regular commercial cleaning products in winter and not opening windows then you are breathing in a certain amount of synthetic chemicals. With asthma a concern for many parents, we are wise to move to cleaning with edible ingredients. I also love opening our windows regularly- the ultimate outdoor scent, rather than the type in a can!

Remember, just a few sprays a day of any toxic cleaning or fragrance products adds up. Some of the toxins you are exposed to on a daily basis are excreted relatively quickly. Yet, as Bruce Lourie and Rick Smith found in their book *Slow Death by Rubber Duck*, daily use of cleaning sprays, antibacterial soaps and other synthetic chemical products means that we are constantly exposed.[187] These toxins can also be absorbed through the skin and what comes through our skin ends up in our blood stream. Scientists believe that most people on the planet now have many potentially toxic compounds in their blood.[188]

Solutions

Leave conventional, heavily-marketed, cleaning products on the shelf.

- **Opt for baking soda.** The cleaning possibilities are endless and effective. You can clean sinks, showers, baths, loos, taps, smelly tennis shoes and mirrors to a sparkling shine. (Well, your tennis shoes won't shine but the rest might!)
- **Buy a genuine essential oil** like lemongrass, lemon or orange and add a drop to your cleaning, particularly if you want an up-lifting smell having cleaned.
- **Open the windows every day,** even just for ten minutes, to get the fresh air circulating. The quality of the air in our homes is just as important as the quality outside. We need fresh air!
- **Get moving whilst cleaning.** Scrubbing floors or vigorously cleaning windows may help detox your body—you are moving and stimulating the lymphatic system. Toxins found in our environment that we are exposed to can get stored in our body fat[189] so it is not just what we eat that may affect your thighs. Remember that the lymphatic system works when stimulated by exercise, so

moving vigorously when you are cleaning the house might be a free gym workout with a clean house at the end!

- **Avoid store bought air fresheners.** These contain synthetic chemicals which are considered toxic, including phthalates. Essential oils work well and have therapeutic benefits for mind and body.

- **Make a paste of baking soda and Castile soap** for your dirty oven or cooker hob. Be sure to use a triclosan–free scrubbing pad. Some oven cleaners can be quite toxic. Baking soda works just as well; leave a layer of the baking soda paste on the dirt and grime for 30 minutes. Rinse off with water. Your arms will enjoy the work out and you'll have a clean oven or hob.

- **Stubborn burnt food** can be removed easily with some of the all purpose cleaner. Put a generous squirt in the dish, some hot water, scrub it about and leave for an hour, or two, or overnight. In the morning the pan will be easy to clean. Far nicer than a spray with heaven-knows what in it!

- **Soap nuts** are a fruit which, as odd as it sounds, have soap-like qualities. They can clean your laundry and I've made a surface cleaner by adding hot water to a few soap nuts.

Save money, lessen your body burden & be fish friendly!

Opting for safer household cleaners will likely save money and reduce your toxic body burden, something all radiant women are wise to do. It will reduce the impact on the water downstream; remember that what we wash down the drain winds up affecting someone else.[190] There is little to beat scrubbing with soap and water and using some elbow grease! (See Appendix for alternatives to household cleaners containing triclosan.)

How to Make...

All Purpose Cleaner

INGREDIENTS:
150g baking soda
50mls Castile soap
50mls boiled water – optional
A dash of glycerin – available at most chemists (drug stores)
An old plastic sauce bottle or a plastic tub to store the cleaner

METHOD:
Combine all the ingredients into the plastic bottle; put the lid on.
Give a jolly good shake.

Use as you would any other all-purpose cleaner. It really is that simple!

If you like a "smell" to associate with cleaning then add up to ten drops of lemon essential oil. That will give a hint of freshness without being over-powering.[191]

Virtuous Vinegar

Vinegar is another non-toxic substance to use for cleaning, as it is acidic.[192] I have used it effectively in our house for mould and I believe it is somewhat anti-bacterial. Don't let the reasonable price of vinegar fool you—the uses are nothing short of miraculous.

Cleaning the inside of the fridge and oven is safe with a vinegar and water solution. The grease on the stovetop or exhaust fan grid can be wiped away with a vinegar-soaked cloth as vinegar cuts through grease.[193]

Vinegar is brilliant for cleaning windows and mirrors in the home and car—just dry with newspaper to stop any streaks. To clean plastic garden furniture, mix one tablespoon of vinegar to one gallon of water, then wipe down with a cloth and leave to dry in the sunshine.

Then you can soak up the spring sunshine with a cup of tea from your newly cleaned kettle. Vinegar effectively de-scales the kettle—just fill the kettle a quarter full with vinegar and a little water, boil and leave to cool, scrub with a cloth if grubby. Be sure to boil at least two full kettles of water (and discard) before making tea, or it will taste really odd. *Trust me* on this one!

I use vinegar in a spray bottle and use with a cloth to say goodbye to mould and mildew in the shower, get rid of lime scale around taps and remove stains in the toilet bowl. Remove soap scum from shower doors by wiping down with a damp cloth sprayed with vinegar. However, do not use vinegar on marble surfaces!

Good Germs, Bad Germs

You now have many ways to clean your home without using synthetic chemicals. Before we leave this topic, I must touch on the popular trend of antibacterial soaps, gels washes and sprays. As I mentioned, in the food section, where we talked about beneficial bacteria for the gut; we *need* bacteria. Not all bacteria are beneficial but I think once again marketing and advertising have led us to believe that the threat from bacteria is far more serious than it really is. I am not sure all this bug-bashing is wise.

Years ago, I thought antibacterial and antimicrobial products were better and bought them. It may surprise you to know that I never stopped to think if antibacterial soap was wise. It appears it wasn't! In 2000, the chair of the American Medical Association said, "There is no evidence that they do any good and there is reason to suspect that they could contribute to a problem by helping to create antibiotic-resistant bacteria."[194]

In 2009, the Canadian Medical Association called on the Federal Government to ban antibacterial household products because of fears they cause bacterial resistance.[195] Vancouver Coastal Health (VCH) advises "not to use antibacterial soap, as using antibacterial hand soaps and antibacterial household cleaners can lead to antibiotic resistance".[196]

Perhaps we all have a duty to stop using antibacterial products to protect each other. Have you ever considered how many antibacterial products you use? Triclosan is a popular ingredient today. While it might sound harmless enough, don't be fooled—it was first registered as a pesticide in 1969.[197] Also, triclosan can mimic hormones and has estrogenic qualities.[198] Unless you're vigilant, daily exposure to triclosan is quite likely as it is found in over 1,600 cosmetic products in Canada, including deodorants, face creams, body lotions, fragrances and shampoos.[199]

What Is Triclosan?

Triclosan is used as a preservative and to stop the growth of bacteria in personal care and household products.[200] It has been studied a great deal recently and the findings are concerning, not least for bio-accumulation. This means the more triclosan you use the more it collects in either our body and or the environment. According to Bruce Lourie and Rick Smith, in *Slow Death By Rubber Duck,* unlike phthalates and bisphenol A, which stay in the body for only a few hours, triclosan sticks around for several days.[201] Since many people are exposed to triclosan on a daily basis through their antibacterial soap, deodorant or toothpaste they are constantly exposed. Studies suggest we should be particularly cautious using triclosan in toothpaste.[202]

Where to find triclosan:

- Antibacterial soap – Triclosan is often listed as an *"active* ingredient"
- Antibacterial household sprays
- Toothpaste – Colgate Total® has 0.03% triclosan
- Dishwashing soap (washing up liquid)

The EU says triclosan is safe to use but in *small doses*.[203] What about small cumulative doses from your soap, toothpaste and dishwashing soap? Doesn't that add up?

Triclosan has been on the non-toxic radar for a number of years and fortunately now the Canadian Government is toying with the idea of deeming it toxic to the environment.[204] This is great news and I hope in the future it will mean we see far fewer products containing triclosan on our supermarket shelves.

. . . .

Personally I think we are wise to avoid triclosan altogether, considering the "precautionary principle".

. . . .

Remember for many years cigarettes were deemed safe; it is only now, many years later, that science has shown us they are detrimental to our health. What will we discover about triclosan in years to come? Only time will tell.

Perhaps you think you only come into contact with a small dose of triclosan in toothpaste or washroom soap. My concern is that a small dose, up to the legally allowed limits,[205] may be calculated by one manufacturer but what about the person using numerous products with triclosan, including antibacterial spray soap five times a day, toothpaste or a dish cloth impregnated with triclosan. Surely they could be exposing themselves to more than a small dose by using all three products, which may contain the maximum legally allowed dose.

This cumulative effect is what concerns me and I am not alone in this. I know that triclosan is showing up in our water supplies and more alarmingly in our soil.[206] The impact of this synthetic chemical anti-bacterial agent is not fully known but we do know that it undergoes photo-transformation in water to form dioxin[207]—a cancer-causing substance.[208]

Why do we seem remarkably reluctant to act when we know enough to warrant action? The United States Centers for Disease Control and Prevention found triclosan present in the urine of 75 percent of Americans over the age of five.[209] I think we're wise to avoid triclosan in toothpaste, soaps and washing up liquids. Whilst there will always be those who say that what is in the market place is safe, I feel we are wise to adopt the precautionary principle

I avoid triclosan in our home but I can't tell what ingredients are in a washroom at an airport or library. I therefore carry a little bottle of Castile soap—easy to do and most of the time it saves me from using unknown soaps. I like Dr. Bronner's handy little soap, the 59ml bottle—it fits in a handbag and is easily refilled from a larger bottle.

Some companies have removed triclosan from their products but have replaced it with its cousin triclocarban,[210] which also has antibacterial properties and is reported to be "more abundant in freshwater environments" than the often-studied triclosan.[211] This is another reason that reading labels is very important!

There is little doubt our personal care and household habits have wide-reaching effects. Perhaps it is time to quit the unnecessary anti-bacterial habit once and for all? You can enjoy a clean, safe home without buying into all the antibacterial marketing that is out there. New products arrive on shop shelves all the time, yet as old fashioned as I sound; very often the older, simple methods are still the best.

GIVE IT A GO

- Check your personal care product labels and avoid antibacterial items as much as you possibly can. Soap and water works well!
- Tell your friends to look out for triclosan. Our water is a precious resource; let's keep it that way.
- Consider making your own household cleaner, it is really a lot easier than you might think! It may well save you money, too.
- Use essential oils to fragrance your home rather than air fresheners. Avoid in-car air fresheners as well!
- Open windows daily to get air circulation in your home.
- If you don't have some already, buy some pot (potted) plants; they look lovely and clean the air at the same time.

CHAPTER 12

. . .

Bringing It All Together

. . .

"Happiness is simply the ability to fully appreciate whatever is happening now."[212]

I have shared a LOT of information with you in *The Radiant Woman's Handbook*. I really hope it hasn't been too daunting to read! I have aimed to make it digestible but some things are quite complex. I trust you will take a few points from it to inspire and encourage you to make a change or two.

Please do not worry if it all seems overwhelming; that's okay. Put the book back on the shelf and go and have a cup of tea. By now you know, I love a cup of tea and taking a break after learning new information can actually help you remember it better. Dr. Lila Davachi, an assistant professor in the Department of Psychology and Center for Neural Science at New York University, says, "Taking a coffee break after class can actually help you retain that information you just learned".[213] So be sure to put *The Radiant Woman's Handbook* down, make yourself a "cuppa" and just look out of the window and relax.

Whilst I have put all this information in a book, it took over a decade for me to implement many of the strategies here and adopt them as part of my "normal" life and I am still learning. I began in 2000 and therefore you should not expect to suddenly change everything at once. Remember what I said at the beginning about a canoe turning at sea? It takes time.

This book is about "out with the old" (well, not that old; most of it has been introduced in the last 50 years) and "in with the new" (which often isn't new but actually old traditional ways). This is "new old learning" if you like. It's what your great-grandmother might have known but didn't tell you.

This book is about less stuff, less busy-ness, fewer distractions and more conscious living, more radiance, more simplicity, more awareness and free time and energy to live the life you were born to live. Life is the here and now, not tomorrow when you have X, Y and Z but now.

. . . .

**Please do not let your past,
whatever that may include,
dictate your future.**

. . . .

You are too precious to live a life regretting what you have done (or haven't done) and what could have been.

Take hold of the essential fact that each new day as the sun rises is a new beginning. It is a new chance to live a radiant day and make your whole life radiant. Our thinking can get stuck like a record player (showing my age as I had a very smart record player growing up!) and go round and round playing the same tune. Sometimes that tune is easier to stick with than changing the record or CD but as challenging as it may seem, changing tune is often worth it.

As I mentioned at the beginning, the main way to succeed is not necessarily do it all at once. Think how you learn to ski; you do not (I hope) hurtle down a black run knowing nothing about choosing terrain, edging, stopping or balancing? No! So, looking after yourself is no different. See what one thing resonates most with you and consider altering that. Then begin to see what else appeals and take it gradually.

As you weed out the synthetic chemicals from your life, you may find you use less. I don't need seven different cleaning products, baking soda and soap work. I don't need serums for this and potions for that; jojoba oil works. I don't want endless new gadgets; clutter is something I am clearing not collecting!

Remember, what has worked for me may not for you. We are all different and life is a journey. My opinion is just that: mine. You can put this book back on the shelf and never again give it a moment's thought. That might work for you and if that is what suits you, I truly wish you a long, happy and joyful life. However, I wrote this book knowing there will be those who will enjoy reading it and over the years they might make some positive, radiant changes.

Time heals. So take time to heal; saying nice things about yourself is wise. Learn what will suit you and use your own body's wisdom to decide where to start. That is precisely why this book is laid out the way it is, giving you pointers but not saying only to do it this way. You are an individual. I know you are intelligent and resourceful enough to make your own decisions. I would just urge you to use discernment and wisdom to decide what is best. Sadly, many in the medical profession are keen on beautifully boxed pills rather than suggesting a small dietary tweak, taking a brisk walk or seeking the wise counsel of an older person in your community.

Having read my book, be kind to yourself. Please do not beat yourself up that you did not know this stuff earlier. Perhaps you, like me, used perfumes for years, drank soya milk, used fragranced washing powders and said "I'm a failure"—and you now wonder, "How I could have been so silly?" I certainly felt like that but over time I realised being regretful or unkind to myself does no good. Forgiving and letting the past go is truly the only way to enjoy living fully immersed in the moment of now, today. "Though your sins are like scarlet, they shall be as white as snow" (Isaiah 1:18).

What that means is today you can forgive yourself; let God forgive you and move on anew, white as snow for the rest of your life. Perhaps you say, "Yes, Joanna, but that's impossible". Well, sorry; I do not think it is; you can have a renewed life, Starting today. Pretty exciting stuff? I think so!

So, forgive yourself and start living today. Renew and reclaim your joy and radiance. They are yours to claim. Will you grab them?

I hope that this book might encourage you to take a daily brisk walk, spend time conversing with positive people, let go of things that no longer serve you, read ingredients labels, and perhaps prioritise a good night's sleep. Maybe it will encourage you to start a new path or merely no longer buy antibacterial soap. If that is the case know that that makes me very happy.

Reading labels, eating good food, resting, walking, laughing, loving and looking into the eyes of those around you is a very radiant place to start. Buying less stuff is another positive first step. Any of these steps you take make my writing this book worth it. I wrote this book to have a positive impact on your life and our beautiful world.

I also hope reading this book will encourage you to stop once in a while and just look around. Life is actually pretty incredible; that a hummingbird flies all the way from Mexico to my garden in cold British Columbia just astounds me. Have you seen a hummingbird?

They are tiny yet God made them so resilient that their minuscule little wings can flap all the way north. I am not suggesting you get all Pollyanna on life but stopping once in a while to just appreciate what is happening now can have a remarkably calming effect.

This book is the result of over a decade of my life, trial and error, reading oodles of long overly-scientific documents and hopefully distilling the information into a format that is relatively easy to understand. This trial and error is often the way life is—a journey, not all flower-strewn pathways. There are some twists and turns and yet if you only get one thing from this book, that is to **love yourself.**

Being radiant comes from liking who you are and trusting that all is in hand. Think back to how powerful your words are and notice how you speak about yourself, your body, your life, your future. Words do matter.

I know that all will be well, regardless of how the world may seem. You are more resourceful than you give yourself credit for. Celebrate being you! Every little bit does count so if you start enjoying your food and not saying negative things about your body then that is a huge step - not every woman does that!

Step out into the world knowing that you are wonderfully made, just the way you are meant to be. None of us are perfect (it's just airbrushing that makes us think we can be) so simply be you and enjoy the experience.

To enjoy today you have to let go of your grip on the past and trust that the future will be good, it will be.

· Endnotes ·

1. Quote taken from Sherry Turkle's website. Accessed 11th January 2013 http://alonetogetherbook.com/
2. Amy Slater Flinders University study 'Poor Body Image Linked with Facebook Time' http://blogs.flinders.edu.au/finders-news/2012/02/21/poor-body-image-linked-with-facebook-time/
3. Chapman, Gary D. *The Five Love Languages: How to Express Heartfelt Commitment to Your Mate*. Chicago: Northfield Pub, 1995. Print.
4. *The Four Agreements* published by Amber-Allen Publishing, 1997. Print.
5. Ted Talk: Dan Gilbert: The Surprising Science of Happiness http://www.ted.com/talks/dan_gilbert_asks_why_are_we_happy.html
6. Gratitude influences sleep through the mechanism of pre-sleep cognitions. Wood AM, Lloyd, Joseph S and Atkins S. School of Psychology, University of Manchester. http://www.ncbi.nlm.nih.gov/pubmed/19073292
7. Emmons Robert A. *Thanks! How the science of gratitude can make you happier.* New York. Houghton Mifflin Company, 2007. Page 33 Print.
8. Mike Wilson quote.
9. Study: Insomnia. Stats Canada. 16th November 2005. http://www.statcan.gc.ca/daily-quotidien/051116/dq051116a-eng.htm
10. Steven W, Lockley and Russell G. Foster, *Sleep: A Very Short Introduction,* Oxford University Press, Oxford, UK: March 2012. Print.
11. Dr. Raymonde Jean, M.D. Director of Sleep, St Lukes Roosevelt Hospital Center, in New York. http://www.huffingtonpost.com/2011/02/02/sleep-health-benefits-_n_817803.html#slide=234465
12. Steven W, Lockley and Russell G. Foster, *Sleep: A Very Short Introduction,* Oxford University Press, Oxford, UK: March 2012. Print.
13. Ibid

14. The Big Sleep: Canada's Dangerous Love Affair with Tranquilizers. http://www.vancouversun.com/health/sleep+Canada+dangerous+love+affair+with+tranquillizers/6924323/story.html

15. A serving of gratitude may save the day. John Tierney. New York Times. http://www.nytimes.com/2011/11/22/science/a-serving-of-gratitude-brings-healthy-dividends.html?_r=0

16. Laura Joahannes, 'Can Lavender Help You Get to Sleep', by Laura Johannes. *Wall Street Journal*. August 24th 2010.

17. Morning exercise may help sleep. NBC News. http://www.nbcnews.com/id/3541400/ns/health-fitness/t/morning-exercise-may-help-sleep/#.URnmSug1aXc accessed 2/11/13

18. Intensive mobile phone use affects young people's sleep: University of Gthernbery, Sahlgrenska Academy, accessed April 2012 http://www.sahlgrenska.gu.se/english/news_and_events/news/News_Detail/intensive-mobile-phone-use-affects-young-people-s-sleep.cid1069245

19. Can tablet screens disrupt sleep? Guardian newspaper 11th September 2012, accessed 29th January 2013. http://www.guardian.co.uk/technology/reality-check/2012/sep/11/can-tablet-screens-disrupt-sleep

20. F.luxTM Better lighting for your computer. http://stereopsis.com/flux/

21. City life it's like jetlag. Roger Highfield. The Daily Telegraph. 27th January 2007. http://www.telegraph.co.uk/science/science-news/3350660/City-life-Its-like-jet-lag-say-scientists.html

22. Ober, Clint, Sinatra, Stephen T and Zucker, Martin. *Earthing The most important health discovery ever?* Laguna Beach. Basic Health Publications. 2010. Print.

23. ibid

24. Earthing: Health implications of reconnecting the human body to the earth's surface electrons. Gaétan Chevalier, Stephen T. Sinatra, James L. Oschman, Karol Sokal and Pawel Sokal. J Environ Public Health. 2012; 2012: 291541.

25. Rehan, Kelly, M. reviewed by Robert M. Sargis, M.D., Ph.D. An overview of the adrenal glands: beyond fight or flight. 30th November 2012. http://www.endocrineweb.com/endocrinology/overview-adrenal-glands

26. Dr. Matsuro Emoto. http://www.masaru-emoto.net/english/emoto.html

27. Dr. Batmanghelidj quote accessed January 2013 http://www.watercure.com/yourbodysmanycriesforwaterhardcover.aspx

28. Tea and coffee 'protect against heart disease'. 18th June 2010. http://www.bbc.co.uk/news/10350373

29. Devine A, Hodgons JM, Dick IM, Prince RL. Tea drinking is associated with benefits on bone density in older women. http://www.ncbi.nlm.nih.gov/pubmed/17921409

30. Sleep: A very short introduction by Steven W, Lockley and Russell G. Foster published by Oxford University Press, March 2012. Print.

31. Bottled water has become liquid gold. Hamo Forsyth. Money Programme. BBC. http://www.bbc.co.uk/news/business-11813975

32. Bisphenol A. National Institute of Environmental Health Sciences. http://www.niehs.nih.gov/health/topics/agents/sya-bpa/

33. Elsevier (2008, October 3). Six Environmental Research Studies Reveal Critical Health Risks From Plastic. *ScienceDaily*. Retrieved January 28, 2013, from http://www.sciencedaily.com¬ /releases/2008/10/081002172257.htm

34. Environmental Obesogens: Organotins and Endocrine Disruption via Nuclear Receptor Signaling. June 2006. Felix Grün and Bruce Blumberg. http://endo.endojournals.org/content/147/6/s50

35. Endocrine-Disrupting Chemicals: An Endocrine Society Scientific Statement Evanthia Diamanti-Kandarakis. http://edrv.endojournals.org/content/30/4/293.long

36. Joan Gussow quote. http://www.quotegarden.com/cows.html

37. Fat Soluble Vitamins. Baumann C.A. and Steenbock, H. Department of Agricultural Chemisty, University of Wisconsin. 2nd February 1934. http://www.jbc.org/content/105/1/167.short

38. Vitamins and minerals in butter. The Dairy Council, UK. http://www.milk.co.uk/page.aspx?intPageID=379

39. Goucheron, F. Milk and dairy products: a unique micronutrient combination. http://www.ncbi.nlm.nih.gov/pubmed/22081685

40. Butter: Kabara, J J, The Pharmacological Effects of Lipids, J J Kabara, ed, The American Oil Chemists Society, Champaign, IL 1978 pp 1-14.

41. Canada's organic food certification little more than an extortion racket, report says. Adrian Humphreys. 24th November 2012. National Post. http://news.nationalpost.com/2012/11/24/canadas-organic-food-certification-system-little-more-than-an-extortion-racket-report-says/

42. Germany investigates organic egg fraud claims. Gareth Jones. The Scotsman. 26th February 2013.

43. University of Texas, Health Science Center, San Antonio. Press Release: http://www.uthscsa.edu/hscnews/singleformat2.asp?newID=3861

44. Excitotoxins: The taste that kills. Russell L. Blaylock, M.D. published by Health Press, 1997.

45. ibid

46. Alphabetical list of E-numbers. http://www.food-info.net/uk/e/e-alphabet.htm

47. MSG and hydrolysed vegetable protein induced headache: Review and case studies. Alfred L. Scopp Ph.D. http://onlinelibrary.wiley.com/doi/10.1111/j.1526-4610.1991.hed3102107.x/abstract

48. Pollan, Michael. *In Defence of Food*. New York. Penguin Books.2008. Page187. Print.

49. Constant stress puts your health at risk. Mayo Clinic. http://www.mayoclinic.com/health/stress/SR00001

50. Tribole, Evelyn and Resch, Elyse *Intuitive Eating*. New York. St. Martin's Griffin. 2nd edition 2003

51. Daniel, Kaayla *The Whole Soy Story* Newtrends Publishing, Inc.; 1st edition (March 10, 2005) http://drkaayladaniel.com/

52. Endocrine disrupting chemicals Diamanti-Kandrakis et al. 2009. page 2. sent on email from Bruce Blumberg. Ph.D.

53. Cao Y, Calafat AM, Doerge DR, Umbach DM, Bernbaum JC, Twaddle NC, Ye X, Rogan WJ 2009 Isoflavones in urine, saliva and blood of infants—data from a pilot study on the estrogenic activity of soy formula. J Expo Sci EnvironEpidemiol 19:223–2344. Calafat AM, Needham LL 2007. Stated in Endocrine disrupting chemicals. Diamanti-Kandrakis et al 2009. Ibid.

54. UV light turns mushrooms into vitamin D bombs. Ditte Svane-Knudsen. 10th July 2012. http://sciencenordic.com/uv-light-turns-mushrooms-vitamin-d-bombs

55. Dr. Natasha Campbell-McBride. http://gapsdiet.com/INTRO-DUCTION_DIET.html

56. *Gelatin in Nutrition and Medicine* by Nathan Ralph Gotthoffer.

57. Snacking not portion size largely driving U.S. over eating. Anne Harding. CNN Health. 30th June 2011. http://www.cnn.com/2011/HEALTH/06/28/snacking.drives.overeating/index.html

58. Clothing sizes: Dressing Up. The Economist. UK print edition. http://www.economist.com/node/21552262

59. The Obesity Epidemic: too much food for thought? R.C.Davey. http://bjsm.bmj.com/content/38/3/360.full

60. Savoury Snack Market Up While the Economy is Down. Jack Sykes. http://www.keynote.co.uk/media-centre/in-the-news/display/savoury-snack-market-up-while-the-economy-is-down/?articleId=754 accessed 28th February 2013.

61. Reducing obesity and improving diet. Anna Soubry, MP. Policy. UK Government. https://www.gov.uk/government/policies/reducing-obesity-and-improving-diet

62. Cognitive restraint can be offset by distraction, leading to increased meal intake in women. France Bellisle and Anne-Marie Dalix. American Journal of Nutrition. August 2001 vol. 74 no. 2 197-200 http://ajcn.nutrition.org/content/74/2/197.full.pdf+html

63. Frequently asked questions. European Food Information Council. http://www.eufic.org/page/en/page/FAQ/faqid/glucose-fructose-syrup/

64. FDA rejects new name for high fructose corn syrup. http://usatoday30.usatoday.com/money/industries/food/story/2012-05-30/high-fructose-corn-syrup-not-sugar/55291460/1

65. How much sugar do you eat? http://www.dhhs.nh.gov/DPHS/nhp/adults/documents/sugar.pdf

66. Sweet heavens: StatsCan finds average Canadian eats 26tsp of sugar a day. http://www.theglobeandmail.com/life/health-and-fitness/sweet-heavens-statscan-finds-average-canadian-eats-26-tsp-of-sugar-a-day/article600803/

67. Sweet Poison. Why sugar is ruining our health. Victoria Lambert. The Daily Telegraph. 12th April 2013. http://www.telegraph.co.uk/foodanddrink/healthyeating/9987825/Sweet-poison-why-sugar-is-ruining-our-health.html

68. Fermented foods bubble with healthful benefits. Casey Siedenberg. Washington Post. 19th November 2012. http://www.washingtonpost.com/blogs/on-parenting/post/fermented-foods-bubble-with-healthful-benefits/2012/11/19/db70ea76-329b-11e2-9cfa-e41bac906cc9_blog.html

69. The 25 Key reasons you want to dramatically reduce or avoid sugar in your diet. http://bodyecology.com/articles/25_reasons_to_avoid_sugar.php#.UTUlSRkZ9Zo

70. Email correspondence with Randall Zamcheck of Body Ecology. 13th March 2013.

71. *The Probiotics Revolution* by Gary B. Huffnagle, Ph.D. with Sarah Wernick published by Bantam Dell. 2007.

72. ibid

73. University of Michigan Health System. 'The Hygiene Hypothesis: Are Cleanlier Lifestyles Causing More Allergies For Kids?.' *ScienceDaily*, 9 Sep. 2007. Web. 27 Feb. 2013.

74. Preserved lemons and limes page 117. *Real Food Fermentation: preserving whole fresh food with live cultures in your home kitchen.* By Alex Lewin, published by Quarry Books. 2012

75. *Pure, White and Deadly* by John Yudkin and Robert H. Lustig, M.D. introduction. Published by Penguin; Re-issue edition (1 Nov 2012)

76. Nutrition and aging skin: sugar and glycation. F.W.Danby Department of Medicine, Section of Dermatology, Dartmouth Medical School, Hanover, U.S.A.. http://www.ncbi.nlm.nih.gov/pubmed/20620757

77. *The New Home Encyclopedia* edited by Joan Wheeler published by Odhams Press Limited 1931; page 888

78. Frequency of bowel movements and the future risk of Parkinson's disease. Neurology 14th August 2001. R. D. Abbott, PhD, H. Petrovitch, MD, L. R. White, MD, K. H. Masaki, MD, C. M. Tanner, D, PhD, J. D. Curb, MD, A. Grandinetti, PhD, P. L. Blanchette, MD, J. S. Popper, D and G. W. Ross, MD http://www.neurology.org/content/57/3/456.short

79. Bone and vegetable broth. R.A. McCance, W. Sheldon, E.M Widdowson. Archive of Disease in children. 1934 August; 9(52): 251–258 http://www.ncbi.nlm.nih.gov/pmc/articles/PMC1975347/?page=1

80. This recipe is based upon Sally Fallon's recipe in *Nourishing Traditions: Publishing The Cookbook that Challenges Politically Correct Nutrition and the Diet Dictocrats* Published by New Trends Revised and updated 2nd edition, 1st October 1999.

81. Cycling and walking must be the norm for short journeys. BBC News. Nick Triggle. 27th November 2012. http://www.bbc.co.uk/news/health-20499005

82. Effect of physical inactivity on major non-communicable diseases worldwide: an analysis of burden of disease and life expectancy. Dr. I-Min Lee ScD, Eric J Shiroma MSc, Felipe Lobelo MD., Pekka Puska MD., Steven N Blair PED, Peter T Katzmarzyk PhD, for the Lancet Physical Activity Series Working Group. http://www.thelancet.com/journals/lancet/article/PIIS0140-6736%2812%2961031-9/abstract

83. Internet use statistic from Com Score

84. Stand Up For Your Health. Physiologists And Microbiologists Find Link Between Sitting And Poor Health. Science Daily. 1st June 2008.

85. *Sleep: A Very Short Introduction* by Steven Lockley and Russell G. Foster published by Oxford University Press.

86. Canadians confused and conflicted over sun protection products. Lauren Vogel. Canadian Medical Journal. http://www.canadianmedicaljournal.ca/content/182/11/E507.short

87. Nanoscience and nanotechnologies: opportunities and uncertainties. The Royal Society and the Royal Academy of Engineering. July 2004. Page 86. http://www.nanotec.org.uk/report/Nano%20report%202004%20fin.pdf

88. Sunshine and vitamin D: why cloudy skies are bad for our health, Sarah Boseley. http://www.guardian.co.uk/society/2012/may/05/vitamin-d-deficiency-sunlight-health

89. Tomatoes found to fight sun damage. Prof. Mark Birch-Machin, University of Newcastle Upon Tyne. http://www.ncl.ac.uk/cals/about/news/item/tomatoes-found-to-fight-sun-damage

90. Doctors should prescribe gardening, says top physician and Thrive Patron. http://www.thrive.org.uk/news/news/news-259.aspx

91. Multisensory training of standing balance in older adults: I. Postural stability and one-leg stance balance. Ming-hsia Hu and Marjorie Hines Woollacott. http://geronj.oxfordjournals.org/content/49/2/M52.short

92. Why do so few of us know how to breathe properly. Jessica Fellowes. The Daily Telegraph. 27th July 2009. http://www.telegraph.co.uk/health/wellbeing/5901075/Why-do-so-few-of-us-know-how-to-breathe-properly.html

93. Computer Vision Syndrome. American Optometric Association. http://www.aoa.org/x5253.xml

94. (From Chapter IX - The Cause and Errors of Refraction (pg 102) 'The Cure of Imperfect Sight By Treatment Without Glasses'

95. To find a Bates Method practitioner: http://www.seeing.org/teachers/

96. Computer eye strain how to relieve it. Dr. Marc Grossman O.D, L.A.c. http://www.visionworksusa.com/computereyestrain.htm

97. Joy Thompson, email 8th June 2011. Integrated vision therapist. http://seeclearlynaturally.com/

98. Techniques: Palming. The Bates Method. http://www.seeing.org/techniques/palming.htm

99. Techniques: sunning. The Bates Method. http://www.seeing.org/techniques/sunning.html

100. Joy Thompson, email 8th June 2011. Integrated vision therapist. http://www.seeingclearlynaturally.com

101. MELT method quote from Sue Hitzmann on email 18th March 2013.

102. MELT method quote from Sue Hitzmann on email 9th October 2012.

103. MELT method quote from Sue Hitzmann on email 18th March 2013.

104. Contribution of a sedentary lifestyle and inactivity to the etiology of overweight and obesity: current evidence and research issues. Jebb, SA and Moore, MS. http://europepmc.org/abstract/MED/10593524/reload=0;jsessionid=7bAQzBg0K8jZfJTAqggZ.2

105. Gary B. Huffnagle with Sarah Wernick. The Probiotics Revolution published by Bantam Dell, softcover July 2008. (page #62)

106. Bartram's Encylopedia of Herbal Medicine. Thomas Bartram. Robinson publishing Ltd. UK 1998. Page 279

107. ibid

108. Why is body brushing good for my skin. Liz Earle. http://uk.lizearle.com/factsheet-body-brushing

109. ibid

110. Lymphatic breast massage. Daya Fisch. http://breasthealthproject.com/lymphatic-breast-massage.html

111. About breast health. http://essentiallypink.com/s.php

112. Hydrotherapy. Dr. Miriam Mazure-Mitchell. http://www.ndaccess.com/DrMMM/Page.asp?PageID=10

113. Alternating hot and cold water immersion for athlete recovery: a review. Darryl J. Cochrane. http://www.physicaltherapyinsport.com/article/S1466-853X%2803%2900122-6/abstract

114. You sweat but toxins likely stay. Chris Walston. Los Angeles Times. 28th January 2008.

115. The Oil that heals. A physician's successes with castor oil treatments. William A. McGarey, M.D.. Virginia Beach. A.R.E. Press. 1993

116. Pelvic Inflammatory disease. University of Maryland Medical Center. http://www.umm.edu/altmed/articles/pelvic-inflammatory-000124.htm

117. Are You Meeting Your Laugh Quota? Why You Should Laugh Like a 5-Year-Old. Psychology Today. Dr. Pamela Gerloff.

118. Anatomy of an illness as perceived by the patient. Norman Cousins. Bantam books. Page 39.

119. Laughter prescription. William B. Strean, PhD. October 2009. http://www.ncbi.nlm.nih.gov/pmc/articles/PMC2762283/

120. The Science of Laughter. Robert Provine. Psychology Today. 1st November 2000. http://www.psychologytoday.com/articles/200011/the-science-laughter?page=2

121. FDA authority over cosmetics. Accessed March 2013. http://www.fda.gov/Cosmetics/GuidanceComplianceRegulatoryInformation/ucm074162.htm

122. Nanoscience and nanotechnologies: opportunities and uncertainties. The Royal Society 30th July 2004. Page 76.

123. FDA authority over cosmetics. 3rd March 2005. http://www.fda.gov/Cosmetics/GuidanceComplianceRegulatoryInformation/ucm074162.htm

124. General requirements for cosmetics. Health Canada http://www.hc-sc.gc.ca/cps-spc/cosmet-person/indust/require-exige/index-eng.php

125. Stable isotope method for studying transdermal drug absorption: The nicotine patch. Neal L. Benowitz MD, Keith Chan PhD, Charles P Denaro FRACP and Peyton Jacob III PhD. San Francisco, California and Ardsley, NY. http://www.nature.com/clpt/journal/v50/n3/abs/clpt1991138a.html 8th May 1991.

126. Product Testing. Food and Drug administration. Last update 13th June 2012. http://www.fda.gov/Cosmetics/Productand-IngredientSafety/ProductTesting/default.htm

127. Environmental Working Group. Alex Formuzis. Popular lipsticks contain dangerous levels of lead. 8th February 2012. http://www.ewg.org/news/news-releases/2012/02/08/popu-lar-lipsticks-contain-dangerous-levels-lead

128. Dr. Linda Katz. Director of the Office of Cosmetics and Colors. Public meeting: cosmetic microbiological safety issues. 30th November 2011. Department of Health and Human Services. U.S. Food and Drug Administration. Center for Food Safety and Applied Nutrition.

129. United Nations Environment Programme and World Health Organisation. http://www.who.int/ceh/publications/endo-crine/en/ February 2013.

130. Scientists claim phthalates in cosmetics may lead to early meno-pause. Michelle Yeomans. 29th November 2012. Cosmetics Design. http://www.cosmeticsdesign.com/Regulation-Safety/Scientists-claim-phthalates-in-cosmetics-may-lead-to-early-menopause

131. State of the Evidence of Endocrine disrupting chemicals. United Nations Environment Programme and World Health Organisation. February 2013. http://www.who.int/ceh/publi-cations/endocrine/en/index.html

132. Phthalates tied to genital deformities in boys. Our Stolen Future. http://www.ourstolenfuture.org/newscience/oncom-pounds/phthalates/2005/2005-0527swanetal.htm

133. Scents and Sensibility. Globe and Mail. Wallace Immen. 9th April 2010. http://www.theglobeandmail.com/report-on-busi-ness/careers/career-advice/scents-and-sensibility-the-fragrant-workplace/article4314396/?page=all

134. Scent-free policy for the workplace. Canadian centre for occu-pational health and safety. http://www.ccohs.ca/oshanswers/hsprograms/scent_free.html

135. Clearing up cosmetic confusion. Carol Lewis. FDA Consumer Magazine. May 1998, revisions August 2000. http://www.logrog.net/users/lkovach/Aerobics/Articles/Clearing%20Up%20Cosmetic%20Confusion%20%28FDA%20Consumer%20Reprint%29.pdf

136. History of Vaseline® http://www.vaseline.co.uk/Carousel.aspx?Path=Consumer/AboutUs/History

137. Material safety data sheet, propylene glycol. http://fscimage.fishersci.com/msds/19870.htm

138. L'Oreal 2011 Annual Report. http://www.loreal-finance.com/_docs/us/2011-annual-report/LOREAL_Rapport-Activite-2011.pdf

139. L'Oreal to buy back shares after sales rise. 11th February 2013. http://www.reuters.com/article/2013/02/11/loreal-results-idUSL5N0BBGUT20130211

140. Current Issues in Women's Health, an FDA consumer special report. Donna E. Shalala, Ph.D., David A. Kessler, M.D., James A. O'Hara III. January 1994. http://www.ebookdb.org/reading/G71AG625354EG0G02C407F69/Current-Issues-In-Womens-Health--An-FDA-Consumer-Special-Report

141. National Organic Program. United States Department of Agriculture. http://www.ams.usda.gov/AMSv1.0/getfile?dDocName=STELPRDC5068442

142. Organic cosmetics. Food and Drug Administration. September 2010. http://www.fda.gov/Cosmetics/ProductandIngredientSafety/ProductInformation/ucm203078.htm

143. National Organic Program. United States Department of Agriculture. http://www.ams.usda.gov/AMSv1.0/getfile?dDocName=STELPRDC5068442

144. Natural and organic beauty brands are set for a good year. Ina Woitalla. 11th January 2011. http://www.mintel.com/blog/natural-organic-beauty-brands-set-good-year

145. Product Liability- European Union. International Law Office. February 2010. http://www.internationallawoffice.com/newsletters/detail.aspx?g=c19cd19e-6900-450d-8dbb-ad4c5b6c0d17

146. Sandra Steingraber. *Living Downstream*. Cambridge, MA. De Capo Press. 2010

147. 'Plastic micro beads' to be removed from soap http://www.cnn.com/2013/01/07/health/microplastics-soap-unilever/index.html

148. Unilever phasing out microplastics: http://www.unilever.com/sustainable-living/Respondingtostakeholderconcerns/micro-plastics/

149. Schwartz, Mark. Household fragrances may be harming aquatic wildlife, study finds. Stanford News. 29th October 2004. http://news.stanford.edu/news/2004/november3/Perfume-1103.html

150. Sandra Steingraber. *Living Downstream*. Cambridge, MA. De Capo Press. 2010

151. Germ killing chemical from soaps, toothpaste building up in dolphins. Brett Israel. 11th August 2009 Environmental Health News. http://www.environmentalhealthnews.org/ehs/news/triclosan-and-dolphins

152. Perfumes filled with unknown chemicals, group alleges. http://www.ctvnews.ca/perfumes-filled-with-unknown-chemicals-group-alleges-1.511396

153. Not so sexy report. Environmental Defence Canada. http://www.cctfa.ca/site/consumerinfo/FragranceReport_Final.pdf

154. Endocrine disruptors as obesogens. Grün F. Blumberg B. http://www.ncbi.nlm.nih.gov/pubmed/19433244

155. Material Safety Data Sheet: Sodium Lauryl Sulfate. http://www.sciencelab.com/msds.php?msdsId=9925002

156. Toxic Air Fresheners. Natural Resources Defense Council. 22nd August 2011. http://www.nrdc.org/living/healthreports/hidden-hazards-air-fresheners.asp

157. Harmful substances and environmental risks: Phthalates. http://www.cancer.ca/Canada-wide/Prevention/Harmful%20substances%20and%20environmental%20risks/Phthalates.aspx?sc_lang=en

158. Toxic effects of air freshener admissions. Anderson RC and Anderson JH. Anderson Laboratories Inc. Vermont, U.S.A.. Arch Environ Health. 1997 Nov-Dec;52(6):433-41. http://www.ncbi.nlm.nih.gov/pubmed/9541364

159. Experts concerned about dangers of antibacterial products. Globe and Mail. http://www.theglobeandmail.com/life/health-and-fitness/experts-concerned-about-dangers-of-antibacterial-products/article4282875/ August 29th 2009.

160. Triclosan and antibiotics resistance. Official website of the European Union. http://ec.europa.eu/health/opinions/triclosan/en/l-3/3-environment.htm

161. Household Products Database. U.S. Department of Health and Human Sciences http://householdproducts.nlm.nih.gov/

162. Adria Vasil. Marketers can label virtually any product 'organic'. 28 April 2011. http://www.thelavinagency.com/blog-adria-vasil-lousy-labels-marketplace.html

163. Plants used in cosmetics, phytotherapy. Talal Aburjai and Fedah Natsheh. Research 17, 987-1000. (2003). http://www.ncbi.nlm.nih.gov/pubmed/14595575

164. Soules, Marshall. Influence the psychology of persuasion. Chapter 6 Scarcity. http://www.media-studies.ca/articles/influence_ch6.htm

165. Frequently asked questions about magnesium. Natural Calm. http://www.naturalcalm.ca/faq.html

166. Get a clay mask for glowing skin. Ismat Tahseen. Times of India. 17th February 2013.

167. How to use Redmond Clay externally. April 2012. http://www.redmondclay.com/2012/using-redmond-clay-externally/

168. ibid

169. Killed by her hair dye: mother who suffered huge allergic reaction dies after year in coma. 25th November 2012. Daily Mail. http://www.dailymail.co.uk/news/article-2238115/Mother-dies-spending-year-coma-following-collapse-using-home-dye-kit.html

170. The New Home encyclopedia, edited by Joan Wheeler. Published by Odhams Press Limited 1932

171. Fife, Bruce. The Coconut Oil Miracle. New York. Avery. 2004. Page 171.

172. In vitro antimicrobial properties of coconut oil on Candida species in Ibadan, Nigeria. Ogobolu DO, Oni AA, Daini OA, Oloko AP. June 2007. http://www.ncbi.nlm.nih.gov/pubmed/17651080

173. Valerie Ann and Susan Worwood in their book Essential Aromatherapy published by New World Library

174. Neal's Yard Natural Remedies. Susan Curtis, Romy Fraser and Irene Kohler. London. Penguin Arkana. 1997. Page 18.

175. Academy of General Dentistry (2009, July 28). Tooth Gel: Healing Power Of Aloe Vera Proves Beneficial For Teeth And Gums, Too. http://www.sciencedaily.com/releases/2009/07/090717150300.htm

176. ibid

177. Comparison of modified Bass technique with normal toothbrushing practices for efficacy in supragingival plaque removal. Poyato-Ferrera, M, Segura-Egea, P, Bullón_Fernández. 24 November 2005. International Journal of Dental Hygiene.

178. Behind the Label. Pat Thomas. The Ecologist. 5th December 2005. http://www.theecologist.org/green_green_living/behind_the_label/268863/behind_the_label_air_fresheners.html

179. Fragranced consumer products and undisclosed ingredients. Anne C. Steinemann. Department of Civil and Environmental Engineering, Evans School of Public Affairs, University of Washington. http://www.sciencedirect.com/science/article/pii/S0195925508000899

180. Endocrine disruptors and asthma-associated chemicals in comsumer products. Dodson RE, Nishioka M, Standley LJ, Perovich LJ, Brody JG, Rudel RA. Silent Spring Insitute, Massachusetts, U.S.A.. http://www.ncbi.nlm.nih.gov/pubmed/22398195

181. Air freshener; out door scent product information. http://
     householdproducts.nlm.nih.gov/cgi-bin/household/
     brands?tbl=brands&id=19001214

182. Pot plants really do clean indoor air. Ronald Wood, Ralph Orwell,
     Jane Tarran, MAIH and Margaret Burchett, FAIH Plants and
     Environmental Quality Group, University of Technology, Sydney
     http://www.plantcareservices.co.za/downloads/2001_nov2.pdf

183. ibid

184. ibid

185. An Introduction to Indoor Air Quality (IAQ) Volatile Organic
     Compounds (VOCs). Environmental Protection Agency.
     http://www.epa.gov/iaq/voc.html

186. ibid http://www.epa.gov/iaq/voc.html#Health_Effects

187. Bruce Lourie and Rick Smith, *Slow Death by Rubber Duck.*
     Toronto Vintage Canada. 2009.

188. Identification of SARA compounds in adipose tissue. Jon D.
     Onstott, John S. Stanley. 31 August 1989.

189. Environmental toxins, obesity and diabetes, an emerg-
     ing risk factor. Mark Hyman MD. Altern Ther Health Med.
     2010;16(2):56-58.

190. Antibacterials Q&A. Dr. Sarah Janssen on the hazards of hor-
     mone disrupting hand cleaners. National Resources Defense
     Council. 2 November 2011. http://www.nrdc.org/living/
     healthreports/antibacterials-qa.asp

191. This cleaning recipe is adapted from TheSmartMama.com a
     website that has for years forged the way for those wishing to
     live a less toxic life.

192. Heinz all natural cleaning vinegar. http://www.heinzvinegar.
     com/products-cleaning-vinegar.aspx

193. ibid

194. Antibacterial soap may not work. BBC News 16th June 2000.
     http://news.bbc.co.uk/2/hi/health/791934.stm

195. Experts concerned about the dangers of antibacterial products. Jennifer Yang. 21st August 2009. Globe and Mail. http://www.theglobeandmail.com/life/health-and-fitness/experts-concerned-about-dangers-of-antibacterial-products/article4282875/

196. Sneezes and diseases. A resource guide for caregivers and parents. Vancouver Coastal Health. Spring 2008. Page 9. http://www.vch.ca/media/SneezesDiseases.pdf

197. Triclosan facts. Environmental Protection Agency. http://www.epa.gov/oppsrrd1/REDs/factsheets/triclosan_fs.htm

198. The trouble with triclosan, how a pervasive antibacterial chemical is polluting our environment and our bodies. Environmental Defence, Canada. May 2012. Page 7.

199. Preliminary assessment on triclosan. Environment Canada. 2.3.1. Cosmetic Products. http://www.ec.gc.ca/ese-ees/default.asp?lang=En&n=6EF68BEC-1

200. ibid

201. Lourie, Bruce and Smith, Rick. *Slow Death By Rubber Duck*. Toronto. Vintage Canada. 2009.

202. Triclosan- a double edged sword. Orthodontic Cyber Journal). Ajay Kumar, Vidhi Thaker (MSc) and Kamlesh Singh (MDS) May 2011. http://orthocj.com/2011/05/triclosan-%E2%80%93-a-double-edged-sword/

203. Scientific Committee on consumer products. Opinion on Triclosan. 21st January 2009. Page 120.

204. Common antibacterial agent called harmful to environment. CBC News. 30th March 2012. http://www.cbc.ca/news/canada/story/2012/03/30/triclosan-antibacterial-environment.html

205. Preliminary assessment on triclosan. Environment Canada. 2.3.1. Cosmetic Products. http://www.ec.gc.ca/ese-ees/default.asp?lang=En&n=6EF68BEC-1

206. Uptake of Pharmaceutical and Personal Care Products by Soybean Plants from Soils Applied with Biosolids and Irrigated with Contaminated Water. Chenxi Wu, Spongberg, Alison, L., Witter, Jason, D., Fang, Min, Czajkowski and Kevin, P., http://pubs.acs.org/doi/abs/10.1021/es1011115?journalCode=

207. Dioxin Photoproducts of Triclosan and Its Chlorinated Derivatives in Sediment Cores Jeffrey M. Buth, Peter O. Steen, Charles Sueper, Dylan Blumentritt, Peter J. Vikesland, William A. Arnold and Kristopher McNeill http://pubs.acs.org/doi/abs/10.1021/es1001105

208. Dioxins and their effect on human health. World Health Organisation. Fact Sheet No. 225. May 2010. http://www.who.int/mediacentre/factsheets/fs225/en/

209. Antibacterial chemical raises safety issues. New York Times. Andrew Martin. 19th August 2011. http://www.nytimes.com/2011/08/20/business/triclosan-an-antibacterial-chemical-in-consumer-products-raises-safety-issues.html?pagewanted=all&_r=0

210. Anti-bacterial additive widespread in US waterways. Rolf Halden, PhD, PE. John Hopkins Bloomberg School of Public Health. 21st January 2005. http://www.jhsph.edu/news/news-releases/2005/halden-triclocarban-triclosan.html

211. Study suggests active ingredients from personal care is polluting water ways. Cosmetics Design. Simon Pitman. 20th August 2012. http://www.cosmeticsdesign.com/Formulation-Science/Study-suggests-active-ingredients-from-personal-care-is-polluting-waterways

212. Lieberman, Jacob. O.D., Ph.D. Take off your glasses and see. New York. Three Rivers Press. 1995

213. Coffee breaks and screen breaks aid memory. Daily Telegraph. 28th January 2010. http://www.telegraph.co.uk/health/health-news/7084270/Coffee-breaks-and-screen-breaks-aid-memory.html

· Bibliography ·

Abehsera, Michael. *The Healing Power of Clay*. New York. Citadel Press. Kensington Publishing Group. 1977.

Baker, Nena. *The Body Toxic*. New York. North Point Press. 2009.

Bartram, Thomas. *Bartram's Encylopedia of Herbal Medicine*. London. Robinson Publishing Ltd. 1998.

Bertherat, Therese and Bernstein, Carol. *The Body Has Its Reasons*. Rochester, VT. Healing Arts Press. 1989.

Blaylock, Russell. *Excitotoxins*. Santa Fe. Health Press. 1997.

Bragg, Patricia and Paul. *Apple Cider Vinegar*. Santa Barbara. Health Science. 2008.

Carlson, Richard and Bailey, Joseph. *Slowing Down to the Speed of Life*. New York. Harper Collins. 1997.

Cloud, Henry and Townsend, John. *Boundaries*. Strand Publishing. 2000.

Cousins, Norman. *Anatomy of an Illness*. New York. Bantam Books. 1979.

Curtis, Susan, Fraser, Romy and Kohler Irene. *Neal's Yard Natural Remedies*. London. Penguin Arkana. 1997.

Enig, Mary and Fallon, Sally. *Eat Fat, Lose Fat*. New York. Hudson Street Press, Penguin Group. 2005.

Fallon, Sally. *Nourishing Traditions*. Washington, D.C. New Trend Publishing. October 1999.

Fife, Bruce. *The Coconut Oil Miracle*. New York. Avery, a member of Penguin Group. 2004.

Gotthoffer, Nathan Ralph. *Gelatin in Nutrition and Medicine*. Great Lakes Gelatin Company. 2011. Kindle edition.

Huffnagle, Gary, B. with Wernick, Sarah. *The Probiotics Revolution*. New York. Bantam Dell. 2008.

Lockley, Steven W. and Foster, Russell, G. *Sleep: A very short introduction.* Oxford. Oxford University Press, March 2012.

Lourie, Bruce and Smith, Rick. *Slow Death By Rubber Duck.* Toronto. Vintage Canada. 2009.

Malkan, Stacy. *Not Just a Pretty Face.* Gabriola Island. New Society Publishers 2007.

McGarey, William. *The Oil That Heals.* Virginia. A.R.E Press 1993.

Meyer, Joyce. *Change your words, Change your Life.* New York. Faith Words 2012.

Meyer, Joyce. *Eat the Cookie. Buy the Shoes.* New York. FaithWords, Hachette Book Group 2010.

Miguel- Ruiz, Fon. *The Four Agreements.* California. Amber-Allen Publishing. 1997.

O'Connor, Siobhan and Spunt, Alexandra. *No More Dirty Looks.* Cambridge, MA. Da Capo Press. 2010.

Ober, Clint, Sinatra, Stephen and Zucker, Martin. *Earthing.* Laguna Beach, CA. Basic Health Publications. 2010.

Rosas, Carlos and Rosas, Debbie. *The Nia Technique.* Portland. Broadway 2004.

Shapiro, Mark. *Exposed.* White River Junction, VT. Chelsea Green Publishing 2007.

Steingraber, Sandra. *Living Downstream.* Cambridge, MA. Da Capo Press Ltd, 2010.

Uliano, Sophie. *Do It Gorgeously.* New York. NY. Hyperion. 2010

Wheeler Joan (editor). The New Home Encyclopedia. England. Odhams Press Ltd. 1932.

Worwood, Valerie Ann. *The Fragrant Pharmacy.* Bantam Books. New York. 1992.

Worwood, Valerie-Ann. *The Fragrant Mind.* Novato, CA. New World Library. 1996.

· Appendix ·

The following is a selection of skin care, household products and real food resources. When using these companies please mention where you read about them—they apparently like to hear that sort of thing!

. . . .

FOOD — A DIFFERENT PERSPECTIVE:

. . . .

180DegreeHealth. Matt Stone is one of my favourite food writers. Matt's no-nonsense, rather cheeky approach is refreshing if you are fed up with diets!
www.180degreehealth.com

Natural Food Finder. A guide to find natural food resources in the UK. www.naturalfoodfinder.co.uk/

Red23.co.uk. Provides a great range of products including cod liver oil, non-toxic skincare, coconut oil and fermented foods.
www.red23.co.uk

Weston A. Price Foundation. Discusses 'real' food and have an annual conference. There are chapters around the world.
www.westonaprice.org

Learn about E-numbers. This is a brilliant website created by Wageningen University in the Netherlands.
www.food-info.net/uk/e/e-alphabet.htm

Laverstoke Park. Fabulous farm shops in Hampshire and Twickenham, England. I love their buffalo milk!
www.LaverstokePark.co.uk

Go Bio Food. www.gobiofood.com/ in Canada.

Great Lakes Gelatin.

  In the U.S.A.: www.greatlakesgelatin.com/consumer/index.php

  In the UK sold by Pure Body Balance. www.purebodybalanceshop.co.uk/Great_lakes_Gelatin_s/60.htm

SKIN CARE PRODUCTS:

Please consider signing the Just Beautiful Campaign pledge: JustBeautiful.ca

My choice of yummy skin care.

Absolutely Pure. British-made shampoo, cleansers and more. www.AbsolutelyPure.com

Akamuti. Soaps, oils and butters made in Wales. www.akamuti.co.uk

Akoma Skincare. Shea butter products. www.akomaskincare.co.uk or in the U.S.A. www.akoma.com

Alaffia. Shea butter products. www.alaffia.com

Ann Marie Gianni skin care. Organic skin care using herbs & spices. Made in America. I like their anti-aging serum! www.Annmariegianni.com

Bare Organics. For baby products and deodorants. Made in Canada. www.bareorganics.ca

Be Clean Naturally. Soaps, skin balms, toothpaste and simple non toxic products. Hand made in British Columbia, Canada. www.becleannaturally.ca

BioEthique Spa. Located in Vancouver, Canada using products made in France. Lovely facials and non-toxic skin care to buy in store or online. www.bioethiqueorganic.com

Deodorant recipe origination: http://howaboutorange.blogspot.co.uk/2010/04/how-to-make-your-own-deodorant.html

Delizioso Skin care. Non-toxic skin care with make up. Made in Canada. www.deliziososkincare.com/DeliziosoHome-US.html

Dr. Alkaitis. Edible organic ingredients. I love their face masks. www.alkaitis.com

Dr. Bronner's soap. www.DrBronner.com

Essence of Morocco. Argan oil, rose essential oil and Rhassoul clay for the hair. www.esofmo.com/

Golden Path Alchemy Skin Care. Organic ingredients with no nasties. Made in America. www.goldenpathalchemy.com/shop/

Green Sisters. Non-toxic herbal skincare, made in BC, Canada. www.greensisters.ca

Handmade Naturals. British-made clay shampoo, balms and oils. www.HandmadeNaturals.co.uk

Hedd Wyn Tamanu. Tamanu nut oil is nourishing for the skin. www.wildtamanuoil.com/

Helena Lane skincare. Organic oil cleansing and serums. Made in British Columbia, Canada. www.helenalane.com

Herbalix Restoratives. For deodorants made in America. www.herbalix.com

Honey Girl Organics skin care made from honey, propolis and clay. www.HoneyGirlOrganics.com

InLight Organic Skincare. Organic products, made in England. www.inlight-online.co.uk/

Kootenay Soap. Soaps made in Canada. www.Kootenaysoap.com

La Bella Figura Beauty. For argan oil face serums and face masks. www.labellafigurabeauty.com/

Miessence. Created by Organic and Natural Pty Ltd, Australia. A superb deodorant, and a baking soda toothpaste. Available online at www.miessence.com

MOOM organics. Remove hair naturally with sugar. Really effective using edible ingredients. Made in BC, Canada. www.Moom.com

MudPuddle. Clay hair wash made in Canada. www. MudPuddle.ca

Nature's Aid. Aloe vera gel with essential oils. Canadian made. www.naturesaid.ca

Neal's Yard Remedies. I love their Wild Rose Beauty Balm. Made in England. www.nealsyardremedies.com

Niko Cosmetics. Certified organic skin care made in Canada. Canadian store: http://storeca.niko.com/ U.S.A. store: http://storeus.niko.com/

NovaScotia Fisherman. Canadian skin care made with kelp. The lip balm is lovely! www.novascotiafisherman.com

OraWellness for Tooth Oil and Bass brushes. www.orawellness.com

Original Purity for genuinely natural skin care made in Canada. www.originalpurityskincare.com/FACE.html

Pure Nuff Stuff. British-made shampoos, soaps and more. www.PureNuffStuff.com

Rocky Mountain Soap Company. Excellent soaps made with essential oils, body butters and sunscreen. Canadian made. www.rockymountainsoap.com/

Sinfully Wholesome. Wild-crafted soaps, oils and soap nuts. www.sinfullywholesome.com

Spiezia Organics. British-made organic ingredient soaps, butters, balms and oil cleansers. www.spieziaorganics.com

Stark Skincare products made in Canada from genuinely natural ingredients. www.starkskincare.com

Terressentials. American-made clay hair wash, body oils and certified organic skincare. www.Terressentials.com

The Organic Pharmacy make lovely skincare which is available worldwide. Their facials are heavenly! www.theorganicpharmacy.com

Tsi-La Natural Perfumery and Organics. Natural perfumes with out synthetic fragrances. www.tsilaorganics.com

. . . .

HOUSEHOLD CLEANING PRODUCTS

. . . .

Berry Plus. An eco-friendly clothes washing liquid that works! A bottle lasts for ages, it's very concentrated. www.berryplus.com/buy-it-now/

BioD. British-made non-toxic cleaning products www.biodegradable.biz/

BioPure. Probiotic cleaner made in Australia. www.miessence.com

Molly's Suds. Non-toxic laundry powder. www.mollyssuds.com/

The Healthy House. A British company selling environmentally friendly and non-toxic products. www.healthy-house.co.uk

Small Planet. Non-toxic cleaning products. Made in Canada. www.smallplanet.ca

EcoHolic. Adria Vasil is a beautiful non-toxic crusader (without a horse). www.ecoholic.ca

Environmental Defence. All things non-toxic and ecological, based in Toronto, Canada. www.environmentaldefence.ca/

Environmental Working Group. Guides on skin care, home care and more. www.ewg.org/consumer-guides

Good Guide. Find out what's in the products you buy. www.goodguide.com/

Gorgeously Green. Sophie Uliano is another English girl, living in North America, talking green. www.GorgeouslyGreen.com

Healthy Child Healthy World. An American website that has a wealth of information for those wishing to clean green and avoid synthetics. www.HealthyChild.org

Household Cleaning Products Database. Created by the U.S. Department of Health and Human Sciences. Easily check the safety of household product ingredients. http://householdproducts.nlm.nih.gov/

MELT Method balls: www.meltmethod.com

Nia Technique. Find Nia and Nia 5 Stages classes in your area. www.nianow.com

The Ecologist. A UK magazine sharing environmental and non-toxic news. www.theecologist.org

The Smart Mama. Non-toxic articles and her book is great! www.thesmartmama.com

The Soft Landing. Discusses avoiding plastics, known toxins and other eco-chic stuff. www.thesoftlanding.com/

· Acknowledgements ·

As with most books, there are many, many people, friends and family who have helped me get to the point of publishing this book.

I am extremely aware that many of my ideas have been developed through meeting some extraordinary and diverse people in my life and having great discussions. I would like to thank everyone who helped shape the thoughts and ideas that allowed this book to be written. In no particular order and if I have forgotten to name you then I am humbly sorry.

To my incredible husband, thank you. You are right; "Just because you are the only one doing it doesn't mean you are wrong". How many times when I felt like binning this book did you make me a cup of tea, give me a hug, cook supper and all was well? Thank you my darling.

To Dad; your visionary thinking inspired me from a young age to think outside the box and even though it isn't easy, to do it anyway!

To my mother; your peaceful spirit and generous nature is inspiring. Thank you for writing me nice letters, cooking me nourishing meals and making me wonderful clothes. Thank you also for instilling in me that a daily walk is vital. It is!

To my sister; thank you for your letters, telephone calls and minibreaks. "Bee Da."

To Granny; for your peaceful way of going with the flow, I hope some rubbed off on me. I love learning from you and hope I look as fabulous as you do at 90 years old.

To Kim; your knowledge and kindness has made the world of difference. Thank you.

To Bruce Lourie for your kind words and encouragement. I smile every time I see rubber ducks in the snow.

To Jennifer Taggart for your straight talking, intelligent views, and for inspiring me that spreading the message of how to live a non-toxic life was vital.

To Uncle John for your encouraging comment one day at lunch about how I am always doing something interesting and making the world a better place; that really struck home. I hope this book enables others to follow suit and do their best to make the world a better place.

To Arlyn for your editing expertise. You have managed to take my convoluted words and make them flow on the page. Thank you for your support, encouragement and prayers. What a joy it was to come to your talk on *Prayer-Saturated Kids* and realise you were also an editor. God moves in wonderful ways.

To Dr. Caren Helbing, PhD, University of Victoria, British Columbia, Canada for sending me your research and sparking an interest in triclosan.

To Dr. Alastair Leake, Head of Project, The Allerton Project, Game & Wildlife Conservation Trust. Thank you for your emails and sharing your experience of triclosan.

To Sally Fallon-Morrell; thank you for your wise words a few years ago; it's ok if someone doesn't agree; it just makes the conversation more fun!

To Loretta; for your brilliant coaching and butt kicks. Thank you for believing in me and telephoning out of the blue.

To Maggie; my sister with a Canadian accent. I am so grateful that we met through Nia and continue to grow our friendship.

To Dr. Susan Jebb, Science Advisor on obesity to the British Government's Department of Health.

To Debbie Rosas, co-creator of Nia; thank you for bringing such a healing, somatic lifestyle practice to the world. I hope that women reading this book will learn "body gratitude".

To Jim and Carole for taking me in and loving me; the year I lived with your family turned my life around. You know how grateful I am.

To Edward Dangerfield for your support and enthusiasm; your wise words have led me to keep going.

To Ashley Pickering (www.ashleypickeringdesigns.co.uk/) for all your design advice - I dread to think how many pages I have printed!

To Camilla; you're one of my best friends I never see. Praise God for the telephone!

To Peter; your practical and encouraging support is wonderful. Despite being here, there and everywhere somehow you find time to answer my phone calls. Thank you for all you do for me.

To Leonie; your heartfelt words inspired me - this is too important a message not to share.

To Philippa; you are inspiring; thank you for encouraging me to be professional and not be afraid to aim for excellence.

To Kerry; you are the most talented massage therapist. Your massages have (alongside tea, Pudgie Pies and walks) enabled this book to be completed. Thank you.

· Index ·

CPSIA information can be obtained at www.ICGtesting.com
Printed in the USA
LVOW13s0254130614

389824LV00003B/34/P